Management

for House Surgeons

WE.

Perioperative Management

for House Surgeons

P.R. Hambly

Senior Registrar in Anaesthetics, Stoke Mandeville Hospital,
Aylesbury, UK

M.C. Sainsbury

Senior Registrar in Anaesthetics, Nuffield Department of Anaesthetics,
Oxford, UK

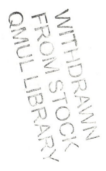
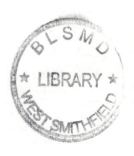

βIOS
SCIENTIFIC
PUBLISHERS

BIOS Scientific Publishers Ltd
9 Newtec Place, Magdalen Road, Oxford OX4 1RE, UK
Tel. +44 (0) 1865 726286. Fax +44 (0) 1865 246823
World-Wide Web home page: http://www.Bookshop.co.uk/BIOS/

DISTRIBUTORS

Australia and New Zealand
    DA Information Services
    648 Whitehorse Road, Mitcham
    Victoria 3132

India
    Viva Books Private Limited
    4325/3 Ansari Road
    Daryaganj
    New Delhi 110002

Singapore and South East Asia
    Toppan Company (S) PTE Ltd
    38 Liu Fang Road, Jurong
    Singapore 2262

USA and Canada
    BIOS Scientific Publishers,
    PO Box 605, Herndon
    VA 20172-0605

Important Note from the Publisher
The information contained within this book was obtained by BIOS Scientific Publishers Ltd from sources believed by us to be reliable. However, while every effort has been made to ensure its accuracy, no responsibility for loss or injury whatsoever occasioned to any person acting or refraining from action as a result of information contained herein can be accepted by the authors or publishers.

The reader should remember that medicine is a constantly evolving science and while the authors and publishers have ensured that all dosages, applications and practices are based on current indications, there may be specific practices which differ between communities. You should always follow the guidelines laid down by the manufacturers of specific products and the relevant authorities in the country in which you are practising.

Typeset by Peter Cox Design Studio, Shillingford, UK.
Printed by Redwood Books, Trowbridge, UK.

CONTENTS

ACTION PAGES

ABBREVIATIONS

A&E	Accident and Emergency
AF	atrial fibrillation
AIDS	acquired immunodeficiency syndrome
APTT	activated partial thromboplastin time
ARDS	adult respiratory distress syndrome
ARF	acute renal failure
AST	aspartate transaminase
AZT	azidothymidine
BMI	body mass index
BNF	British National Formulary
BP	blood pressure
CABG	coronary artery bypass graft
CCU	Coronary Care Unit
CK	creatine kinase
CMV	cytomegalovirus
CNS	central nervous system
CPR	cardiopulmonary resuscitation
CSF	cerebrospinal fluid
CT	computerized tomography
CTZ	chemoreceptor trigger zone
CVA	cerebrovascular accident
CVP	central venous pressure
CVS	cardiovascular system
CXR	chest X-ray
D&C	dilatation and curettage
DDAVP	1-deamino-8-D-arginine vasopression
DIC	disseminated intravascular coagulation
DKA	diabetic ketoacidosis
DNR	'do not resuscitate'
2, 3-DPG	2, 3-diphosphoglycerate
DVT	deep vein thrombosis
ECF	extracellular fluid
ECG	electrocardiogram
EMLA	effective mixture of local anaesthetic
ENT	ear, nose and throat
EPSE	extrapyramidal side-effects
FBC	full blood count
FDP	fibrin degradation product
FFP	fresh frozen plasma
FRC	functional residual capacity
GA	general anaesthetic
GCS	Glasgow Coma Scale
GI	gastrointestinal
γ-GT	γ-glutamyl transferase

GTN	glycerol trinitrate
HAFOE	high airflow oxygen enrichment
Hb	haemoglobin
HBsAg	hepatitis B surface antigen
HBV	hepatitis B virus
HDU	High Dependency Unit
HIV	human immunodeficiency virus
HOCM	hypertrophic obstructive cardiomyopathy
HR	heart rate
5-HT	5-hydroxytryptamine
ICF	intercellular fluid
ICU	Intensive Care Unit
INR	International Normalized Ratio
IPPV	intermittent positive pressure ventilation
ITU	Intensive Therapy Unit
JVP	jugular venous pressure
LA	local anaesthetic
LFT	liver function tests
LSCS	lower segment caesarean section
MAOI	monoamine oxidase inhibitor
MCHb	mean corpuscular haemoglobin
MCV	mean corpuscular volume
MDU	Medical Defence Union
MHA	Mental Health Act
MI	myocardial ischaemia
MO	morbid obesity
MPS	Medical Protection Society
MRSA	methicillin-resistant *Staphylococcus aureus*
MS	multiple sclerosis
MST	controlled-release morphine sulphate
MUGA	multi-gate acquisition
NCEPOD	National Confidential Enquiry into Perioperative Deaths
NIDDMS	non-insulin-dependent diabetes mellitus
NSAID	non-steroidal anti-inflammatory drug
PCA	patient-controlled analgesia
PE	pulmonary embolism
PEEP	positive end-expiratory pressure
PONV	perioperative nausea and vomiting
PTT	partial thromboplastin time
PRN	*pro re nata*
PRV	polycythaemia rubra vera
PT	prothrombin time
SAGM	saline–adenine–glucose–mannitol
SSRI	selective serotonin re-uptake inhibitor
SVT	superventricular tachycardia
TB	tuberculosis

TCRE	transcervical resection of endometrium
TPN	parenteral nutrition
TTO	to take out
TUR	transurethral resection
TURP	transurethral resection of the prostate
U&E	urea/creatinine kinase and electrolytes
UTI	urinary tract infection
VAS	visual analogue scale
VEDP	ventricular end-diastolic pressure
VEDV	ventricular end-diastolic volume
VF	ventricular fibrillation
VT	ventricular tachycardia

PREFACE

This is not a textbook of surgery.

We are anaesthetists. For us, the rectal examination is but a faded memory, and for all we know, cholecystitis could be a Swedish tennis player. If you want to know how to inject haemorrhoids, do not buy this book.

We do, however, retain painful memories of our own dismal efforts as house surgeons. Our lack of experience led us to treat postoperative oliguria as a state of acute frusemide deficiency, postoperative confusion as a sudden shortage of haloperidol. We understood that oxygen was an evil and dangerous drug that should be withheld from patients as much as possible, and if someone said it still hurt after 25 mg of pethidine, we *knew* they were faking.

Our difficulties were in part because of a lack of relevant training, and difficulty in finding relevant information in books. A glance at any surgical text, even most of those aimed at housemen, demonstrates that topics such as analgesia, fluid balance, preoperative preparation, and the interaction of medical illness with surgery, are covered sketchily, if at all.

We have included no surgery in this book. This is most obviously because we don't know any, but also because the house surgeon has constant access to educated opinion on points of surgery, from his or her seniors, or from one of a range of excellent textbooks. When, however, the problem is a breathless patient or postoperative hyponatraemia, useful advice is not so readily available.

Clearly, many aspects of the care of surgical patients cross into a wide range of other disciplines, such as anaesthetics, microbiology, radiology, medicine, intensive therapy, haematology and palliative care. In writing this book, we have tried to collate relevant information from all these specialties.

We have tried to provide as much step-by-step advice as possible, whilst at the same time we acknowledge that medicine cannot be practised from instructions on the back of an envelope. Throughout the text, we have emphasized the importance of the **servo loop** as a tool for guiding management. We believe that the cycle of assessment–therapy–reassessment is the only way to tailor treatment to an individual situation, and is underused. We have included no detailed descriptions of practical procedures like central line insertion, because these should be learnt by real-life demonstration, not from a book.

We hope the result will provide help with those questions to which, at 3 a.m., no-one seems to have the answers.

P. R. Hambly and M.C. Sainsbury

ACKNOWLEDGEMENTS

Much of this book would have been impossible without contributions from: Dr David Butler, consultant in palliative care medicine; Mr Andrew Higgins, consultant urologist; Mr R. Corner, HM Coroner, N. Buckinghamshire; Dr Martin O'Connor, senior registrar in microbiology; and Dr Rebecca Mather, consultant psychiatrist

...well, it wouldn't be impossible, but half of it would be wrong. We also gratefully acknowledge the immeasurable contribution from our wives, Cathy and Claire, for clinical advice, childcare, typing, proof-reading, tea, sympathy, biscuits and patience.

Chapter I.1

COMMUNICATIONS

Chapter I.1

COMMUNICATIONS

KEY POINTS

Please your patients by looking professional, learning their names and explaining everything you do.

Please your defence society by keeping good records and taking consent properly.

Please your colleagues by talking to them in person and in good time.

Please the nurses by using their expertise properly.

Please your consultant by keeping theatres, the anaesthetist and the GPs sweet.

Introduction

Junior surgeons are the interface between the patients and the rest of the surgical team. It is a vital and difficult role. You will be judged more on your communication skills than on any other aspect of your job. Patients will grade your 'bedside manner', and your seniors will base your reference on your smooth running of the firm. This chapter is a collection of hints on communication.

Talking to patients

Names
Always learn the patient's name as a first move, as a common courtesy and to avoid catastrophic confusion. Appear to remember the name; a shifty glance at the head of the bed often helps. If a patient has a rank or title, use it until asked not to. For some generations, the use of Christian names is grossly discourteous. If an elderly lady does not answer to her Christian name she may have forgotten it through disuse, or she might be giving you a lesson in manners.

Dress code
You know perfectly well what doctors are supposed to look like. Sorry, but you have to forget your fashion statement and look the part. This means a tie and a daily shave (especially for the men). A recent survey shows that what patients most like to see is an identifying badge and what they hate most are theatre clogs.

Make time (or pretend to)
Even when you're busy, avoid being curt. Shake hands and sit down. It gives the impression of a longer interview as well as bringing you to eye-level. You will become adept at steering a rambling patient back to the point without appearing rude. It is extremely frustrating to both you and the patient when

you have differing expectations of the interview. Make it clear at the outset what the visit is for (e.g. "I'm here to set up a drip", or "I need to clarify these points in your history"). It is then much easier to get back to the point and to close the interview when the specified task is accomplished.

Chaperones

Essential. Doctors of both sexes need them. Remember that the chaperone is there to protect the doctor, not the patient.

Jargon

Jargon is the secret language that professionals use to intimidate lay persons. It makes you a bore at parties and isn't helpful in talking to patients. If you must use technical terms, translate them for the patient.

Consent

Too much emphasis is put on the *signing* of the consent form. This is only one part of the process of fully informing and consenting. It's a complex subject, but essentially the *minimum* requirement is that the patient is given adequate information to make up his or her own mind about the procedure. This means that alternative treatments, risks, benefits and side-effects must all be covered. It is difficult to know whether to mention rare side-effects, but a side-effect with an incidence of 1% or more is definitely worth discussing. Blood transfusions are worth a specific mention as part of the operative technique; many patients will have questions about AIDS or hepatitis risk (see Chapter II.7).

Stick to what you know when explaining a technique. If asked about specialist stuff (usually about the anaesthetic) just answer that the specialist will be visiting in person. Fill in the form in the presence of the patient, not in advance. Avoid jargon. Use diagrams to explain anatomy and draw them on the back of the form as further evidence that the surgery was discussed in detail. Avoid abbreviations. Add to the text of the form a note that you have talked about side-effects. A useful way of checking that your explanation was adequate is to get the patient to explain the surgery back to you.

Consent is only meaningful if it is given freely. Thus, it must be obtained before pre-medication (although consent should not delay analgesia in an emergency) and before sending the patient to a hostile environment (e.g. the anaesthetic room). You are absolutely not allowed to bully your patients into surgery, even if you have their best interests at heart.

Some other forms of consent deserve a special mention.

Children

The legal age for consent is 16, below this age a parent or guardian is asked to give consent. A guardian may be a relative, a school staff member or a court appointee. The same rules of explanation apply. Older children also have the right to refuse surgery. If a child who fully understands the consequences declines surgery (even if the parent has given consent), you would be on very thin legal ice to proceed. Pass the buck upwards.

Incompetence

Not yours, the patient's. If a patient, through handicap or mental illness, is unable to give fully informed and free consent it may be necessary to ask a guardian (if there is one) to consent on their behalf. The law does not automatically recognize the next-of-kin as a guardian and there is no legal basis for asking a member of the family to give consent for an incompetent patient. Urgent surgery can still be performed for incompetent patients in the absence of consent as long as it is clearly in the patient's best interest and in accordance with accepted medical practice. Most people under psychiatric care are not incompetent; if in any doubt ask for expert help from a psychiatrist. Even if incompetent to give consent, all patients deserve as full an explanation as possible.

Telephone/verbal consent

This is, of course, not a true form of consent at all. It is just another way of communicating with the patient's family. Make a detailed entry in the notes of who you spoke to, the date and time, the explanation you gave and any questions that were asked.

Assumed consent

Patients rendered incompetent (i.e. unconscious) through illness or injury cannot give consent. It is assumed that most rational people would choose to have surgery in these circumstances. Surgery can proceed on the assumption that the patient would have agreed were he able.

Special requests

Some patients request that a specific procedure be avoided. For example, Jehovah's Witnesses often refuse blood transfusion. This is a perfectly reasonable request and must be respected, even to death. Conflict may arise over transfusions for the children of Jehovah's Witnesses. In elective cases, there is time for a full discussion and to seek legal and ethical advice. In an emergency, where a transfusion would be definitely life-saving, most of us would go ahead and transfuse. This decision must be referred to consultant level (see also Chapter II.7).

Advanced directives

Written instructions may be left in anticipation of a time when a person ceases to be autonomous (i.e. loses the ability to make their own decisions). These too should be respected. Occasionally, the advanced directive may disagree with the family's wishes; in this case the former has supremacy. Some people may appoint a representative to enforce their advance directive, this may be a friend or lawyer (or both) but not always a member of the family.

More difficult situations

Dealing with complaints

Complaints are bound to arise. Some of them will be unjustified, but not all. To minimize the fall-out from a complaint you should apologize early. An apology is not an admission of liability. Explain the circumstances of the problem truthfully; for example, most postponements of operations have a perfectly reasonable explanation. Facilitate complaints by referring them up the line to your seniors. Give reassurance that the complaint will not lead to a change in your attitude to the patient (except maybe for the better). Encourage the complaining person to write their version. Document your own version exactly and keep a photocopy. In all but the most minor cases talk to your defence society. Always keep your membership of the MDU or MPS active, you will never regret it.

Giving bad news
This is covered in the Final Chapter.

Talking to families
Families sometimes make difficult requests such as wanting to withhold information from the patient. The patient's interests must always be put first; if he requests information he must be given it. Remember also that families do not have any absolute right to information and that you do have a duty of confidentiality. If the patient wants any information withheld from his family, he does have that right.

Families are very much at risk of receiving conflicting information. To minimize this insist that one family member be nominated spokesperson and channel information through them. It is very helpful to keep a communication sheet to record details of all conversations with the family.

Talking to each other

Talking to other departments
One of your roles as a junior surgeon is liaison between departments. To make a good impression try to make personal visits to other departments whenever feasible. Telephoning is the next best thing. Try to use bleeps as seldom as possible; they irritate people. Make at least a token daily visit to your ITU patients, if only to find out if they are still alive.

When consulting another specialty ask for advice, not services. For instance do not ask an anaesthetist to 'do an epidural', ask for 'help with pain management'. Ask cardiologists for help assessing the heart, don't tell them to do a MUGA scan. The end results are the same, but asking nicely makes the specialist feel more important.

Talking to GPs
It took me painful years to learn this; when a GP wants you to admit a patient, there's nothing you can do to escape it. Accept with good grace and earn yourself a reputation for being helpful. On discharging a patient make sure a brief note leaves with them; the least their GP will need to know is the nature of the surgery, any complications, the drug regime and the follow-up arrangements. It's a little embarrassing for the GP to find out about a death days late and from the relatives. A phone call within the first day of a death should prevent you from shortening your own life expectancy.

Talking to ward staff
Nurses have the power to make or break you as a junior surgeon. Learn their names, treat them with respect and *ask their advice*; they may have 10 times your experience and also know your consultant's idiosyncrasies. Senior nurses

deserve to be called by their titles, especially in formal settings like ward rounds. Nurses' training covers many areas that are a complete mystery to doctors. They can give a lot of help in fields such as organizing discharges and community services, without which your beds stay full. Ward clerical staff can show you a multitude of short cuts through the paperwork and only have to be asked.

Everyone in the hospital has an important job and deserves respect. A white coat is just a practical work garment and not a caste symbol.

Last, but not least, never call a midwife 'nurse'.

Note-keeping

When you make notes, always keep in mind that you are talking to two types of professional: doctors and lawyers. The main reasons for keeping good notes are:

- to record information for others (e.g. on-call staff);
- to refresh your own memory;
- to help formulate your thoughts;
- to protect yourself from litigation.

Good records are always clearly dated and timed, and every page carries the patient's full name and identifying number. Head each entry with the reason for the visit (asked to see, elective admission, operation note, etc.) and follow with history and examination in the usual way. When writing an impression, or giving an opinion, stick within the limits of your training. Do not, for instance, record 'fit for anaesthetic' as you are not qualified to make that judgement and you may look silly in court when giving details of your anaesthetics experience.

You must avoid using any derogatory remarks in the notes. Try substituting 'obese, elderly, talkative' for 'fat old windbag'.

If you put a plan of action at the end of a note, be sure to follow it through. If you talk to a senior, be sure to record the fact, thus neatly passing the buck. There is no point in writing your intention to perform investigations, or even the fact that you have taken samples. All that matters is the results. Put them in the notes, think about them, draw attention to abnormal values.

Finally, at the end of every note, sign your full name. If your writing is like mine, print it as well.

Talking to theatres

Emergencies. Give as much advance notice as possible to both theatre staff and to the anaesthetist of emergency cases. They need time to assess the case and prepare for the patient. However, do not book cases presumptively. At best this wastes everyone's time, at worst it could lead to an unnecessary operation.

If you have a patient whose condition demands urgent surgery, you must contact not only the anaesthetist, but also any surgeons whose cases will be delayed by yours. Theirs may be urgent too.

Elective lists. Creating a list is an art form. There is some debate over whether long cases go at the beginning or end of the list; this is largely the operating surgeon's decision. Where possible try and get the following towards the front of the list:

- children (they don't tolerate waiting well);
- diabetics (to simplify management);
- day-cases (so they can go home).

And put these at the end:
- infected cases (because theatre has to be cleaned out);
- cases needing postop ITU (so transfer time doesn't interrupt the list).

Give thought to availability of surgical equipment. For instance, check that there are enough laparoscopes before booking two laparoscopic cholecystectomies in a row. Don't force frequent changes of operating tables (e.g. from normal to orthopaedic reduction tables).

The written list itself must be carefully prepared to avoid any chance of error. Each patient must be identified by first and last names (in block capitals) and an identifying number. The operations should be written in full, not abbreviated, and the side specified. In many hospitals it is also routine to add the expected duration of the case, requests for special equipment or X-ray, and blood availability. The complete list should be headed with the date, the operating surgeon and the anaesthetist. Identify yourself at the bottom of the list in case of any enquiries.

Submit the list early and, if any changes have to be made, inform theatres, the surgeon and the anaesthetist.

Locals and generals. Traditionally, cases have been listed as LA (local anaesthetics) or GA (general anaesthetics). The convention is that GA cases require an anaesthetist whether he chooses to give a GA or not. If you list a case as LA the anaesthetist will assume that his services are not required.

Cancellations. Cases should be cancelled only when the surgery is not needed (i.e. the pathology has resolved) or when it is not justified (e.g. too great a risk or patient unlikely to survive long enough to benefit). Palliative operations may still be indicated even when the patient is clearly terminally ill. The decision to cancel must be referred to senior staff.

Postponements. Cases should be postponed when it would be dangerous to proceed for logistical or patient-related reasons.

Logistics:
- Think to yourself, is this the right *time* to be operating? Elective lists must not be allowed to creep into the evening and delay emergencies; only emergencies which threaten life, limb or sight should continue after midnight. The fact that your boss might have put too many cases on the list does not justify trying to re-book the last one as an emergency. Like the man said, "your inefficiencies are not my emergencies".
- Do we have the right *people* to be operating? To proceed without adequate numbers or seniority of surgeons, nurses or anaesthetists is dangerous. Nor do personnel function well if denied food and coffee all day.
- Do we have the right *equipment* to be operating? The availability of specialized instruments or cross-matched blood must be checked.
- Are the right *postop facilities* available? Don't start on an elective aneurysm without checking on the bed state in ITU.

Patient factors:
- Is this patient in optimum (not necessarily perfect) condition for surgery? If there is any pathology which can be reversed, time must be allowed to achieve this. Even in very urgent cases there is usually benefit in partial correction of biochemical disturbance and rehydration. Rarely (usually in

severe trauma, ruptured aneurysm, etc.) patients are too ill *not* to have an immediate operation.

Prescriptions

Bad prescribing habits are dangerous for obvious reasons, and also will cause you to be bleeped to come and make alterations. In general, use indelible ink, generic names and capital letters. Try not to use abbreviations for drug names, although some abbreviations are acceptable for doses, timings and route (see below). Red ink is normally used to highlight allergies, and green is used for corrections or recommendations by pharmacy, so avoid using them to prescribe. Where there is any possible source of confusion (e.g. between mg and mcg), clarify by writing 'milligram' or 'microgram' in words. When a course is prescribed (e.g. of antibiotics), be sure to add a stop date.

For some drugs, mostly compound preparations, it is normal to prescribe the amount of drug as the number of tablets. For most other drugs, including liquid preparations, prescribe the amount in grams, milligrams or micrograms of active ingredient. Accepted abbreviations are given in the following tables.

Routes

o. or **p.o.**	oral route
n.g.	nasogastric
s.l.	sublingual
p.r.	rectal
top.	topical
s.c.	subcutaneous
i.m. or **im**	intramuscular
p.v. or **pv**	per vaginam
i.v. or **iv**	intravenous

Any of the more obscure routes (e.g. into the eyes, ears or body cavities) are better written in full to avoid confusion.

Doses

G. or g.	grams. The lower case is preferred
mg	milligram. One thousandth of a gram
mcg	microgram. This form is preferred to the old μg which can be confused with Mg, which would signify either elemental magnesium or a megagram (one metric tonne), neither of which should be given intravenously
T, TT	one tablet, two tablets, etc.
Caps1, Caps2	one capsule, two capsules, etc.
ml or mls	millilitres. Preferred to cm^3 or cc
mmol	millimoles. Usually used to express amounts of ions added to i.v. solutions
mcg/kg/min	Microgram per kilogram of body weight per minute. Used for very powerful substances in infusions (e.g. inotropes)
units	Historically used for biologically derived drugs. Now most commonly for insulin or heparin.
gutt.	gutta. Latin, a drop

Timings

PRN or prn	Pro re nata. As things dictate. Used in the sense of 'if the nurse feels like it'
QID or QDS	Four times per day (but not necessarily at 6-h intervals)
TID or TDS	Three times per day
BID or BD	Twice per day
OD	Once per day
mane	In the morning. This is Latin, not French, and has no accent
nocte	At night. As above
1hrly	At intervals of 1 h
Stat	Immediately

Concentrations

1/1000	One in 1000. Equivalent to 1 mg per ml
% w/v	1% weight per volume equals 10 mg per ml
N. or normal	Only commonly used in 'normal saline'. Equals 0.9% w/v saline

Chapter I.2

PREPARATION OF HEALTHY PATIENTS

PREPARATION OF HEALTHY PATIENTS

KEY POINTS

The reasons for clerking elective cases are:
> To review the surgical pathology and confirm the plans for operation
> To identify problems in general health using clinical skills
> To use this to direct relevant investigations (including cross-matching)
> To review and optimize medical treatments
> To answer questions and gain informed consent
> To establish a rapport with the patient.

Day-case patients need:
> To be carefully selected for medical, surgical and social suitability
> To be assessed to the same standard
> To be consented to the same standard
> To be reassessed before discharge
> To be given information on further care.

Clerking the elective case

Most patients admitted for elective surgery are not only healthy but also have an established surgical diagnosis. Therefore, the clerking process is easily simplified.

The surgical lesion is confirmed by history and examination. Check against the out-patient notes for any changes in symptoms or signs which might alter the indication for surgery. For many operations it is appropriate to mark the site (do this after taking consent).

Conduct a 'systems review' and examination with particular focus on the cardiovascular and respiratory systems. A detailed drug history is vital and may also be a pointer to illnesses which the patient neglects to mention. Record any allergies including those to sticking plaster or iodine. When antibiotics are likely to be used, ask specifically about previous exposure.

Preoperative investigations

These are the bane of the house surgeon's life. The authors of this book fully appreciate that you absolutely **cannot win**. You are guaranteed grief from:
- picky anaesthetists who expect you to either be psychic or possess the FRCA exam;

- homicidal consultant surgeons, who hold you responsible because their cases have been cancelled by picky anaesthetists;
- radiologists, haematologists and chemical pathologists, who will criticize you if you order tests that are not absolutely necessary.

Generally speaking, preoperative investigations can be divided into three groups:

1. *Screening tests* are done on healthy patients for reasons not related to the surgery. Few such tests are necessary. They apply when the risk of *occult* abnormality in a particular group of patients is reasonably high. Examples are:

    ward urinalysis for all patients;
    full blood count for age >60 or gynae patients;
    urea and electrolytes for age >60;
    ECG for age >60 (or younger if major surgery, smoker, etc.);
    chest X-ray for recent immigrants from areas with a high incidence of TB;
    Sickledex test for previously untested patients of Afro-Caribbean origin;
    haemoglobin electrophoresis for those with positive Sickledex.

2. *Tests which are necessary because of the surgical pathology or the nature of planned surgery.* For example:

    full blood count for major surgery, acute abdomen, anticipated significant blood loss;
    urea and electrolytes for major surgery, acute abdomen, vomiting, intravenous therapy, before TURP (for baseline sodium);
    ECG, and in some centres echocardiography, for major surgery;
    chest X-ray for assessment in malignant disease, looking for metastases or pleural effusions, major trauma, major vascular/thoracic surgery;
    cross-matching (see below);
    coagulation studies before surgery for obstructive jaundice.

3. *Tests made necessary by pre-existing illness or its treatment.* This is where most problems arise, and it is the area where omissions are most likely to get your patients cancelled.

    It would require an encyclopaedic knowledge of anaesthesia and medicine to predict what will be required in every case, so the first rule is to anticipate difficult patients and ask advice from the anaesthetist concerned. Advice on preoperative investigations for common medical conditions is given in Chapters I.5–I.13, so refer to that where there is a known diagnosis. Commonly forgotten tests include:

    urea and electrolytes for diuretic therapy;
    ECG for anyone with hypertension;
    C-spine X-ray for rheumatoid arthritis.

Cross-match

Blood products and laboratory time are valuable assets – don't waste them. Preoperative cross-matching depends on many factors, including local preferences and protocols. Opposite is a rough guide to requirements for common operations.

Patients with local inflammation, trauma, connective tissue disease, coagulopathy or invasive tumour are likely to bleed more and require greater cross-match.

Group and save	Cross-match 2 units	Cross-match 4 units	Cross-match 6 units
Need for transfusion unlikely	Need for transfusion likely	Transfusion definite	Transfusion definite
			Check platelet and FFP availability
Expected blood loss 500–1000 ml	Expected blood loss 1000–2000 ml	Expected blood loss 2000–3000 ml	Expected blood loss >3000 ml
Normal preop Hb for : • LSCS • Hysterectomy • TURP • Nephrectomy • Large bowel resection • Vascular fem-pop/carotid • Thyroid • Free-flap	Group 1 patients if low Hb preop (or CVS risk) • Nephrectomy • Joint replacement • Craniotomy • Retropubic prostate • Lobectomy/ pneumonectomy	• Major back, cranial or facial surgery • Major vascular surgery (e.g. aorta) • CABG • Commando or laryngectomy • A.P. resection • Oesophagectomy	• Liver • Pelvis • Bony tumour resection • Thoracic aorta

Day cases

These form an increasing proportion of a surgical team's work. Patients must be carefully selected; contraindications are given in the following table.

Surgical	Social	Patient
Long surgery Likely to need transfusion Expert postop care (i.v. antibiotics) Open body cavity surgery Painful surgery Prolonged immobility	Long distance (>1 h) No phone No adult help No transport	Extremes of age Uncontrolled CVS disease • Angina • BP • Rhythm • Failure • Previous stroke • MI • Claudication Severe respiratory disease (judged by exercise tolerance) Insulin-dependent diabetes Liver disease Renal disease All myopathies Advanced neurological disease

Note: patients with controlled hypertension, asthma or non-insulin-dependent diabetes may be appropriately treated as day-cases.

Successful day-case surgery relies on good communication between the hospital staff, the patient and the GP. A written set of rules is ideal to explain the dos and don'ts to the patients. This should include advice on preop starvation (usually 6 h) and drug regimes (most drugs are continued unchanged, but see Chapter I.3). Postoperatively, patients should be warned to avoid driving, alcohol and using any machinery for 24 h. On discharge, written information should accompany the patient for the GP's benefit. This should include the treatment, the analgesia regime and any plans for further wound-care, stitch removal or follow-up.

All patients must be formally assessed as being fit for discharge; this applies to local anaesthetic cases as well as general anaesthetic cases.

Is the patient fit for discharge?

- Wounds dry
- Patient able to walk; tolerate food and fluid; pass urine
- Stable normal values for vital signs for at least 1 h
- Pain, nausea and vomiting under control
- Social arrangements adequate
- Patient able to understand further instructions

Chapter I.3

PREOPERATIVE RITUALS

Chapter I.3

PREOPERATIVE RITUALS

KEY POINTS

Premeds are desirable to alleviate anxiety, treat pain, reduce the risk of aspiration or prevent some intraoperative problem, but they are rarely essential.

Starvation is essential before elective surgery, whether done under GA or not. Four hours for solids and 2 h for clear fluids have been shown to be safe, but the ethereal logistics of an operating list make such a regimen difficult to implement safely. Most hospitals have a 'nil by mouth after midnight' system. A sip of water to take tablets is perfectly safe, and better than withholding usual medication.

Regular medication, with a few notable exceptions, should always be continued throughout the perioperative period. Exceptions are diabetic medication, anticoagulants and lithium.

Prostheses should be removed if possible to avoid loss or injury. Contact lenses are particularly important. The need to remove teeth is being re-appraised. Cover all rings, etc., with tape to avoid diathermy burns.

Premeds

The premed is part of the anaesthetic technique, and it is the anaesthetist's responsibility to write it up at the time of the preoperative assessment.

The choice of premed is highly individual. Some anaesthetists prescribe the same for everyone, some tailor the agent to the situation, and some prescribe none at all. Therefore, if the anaesthetist hasn't written a premed, and the patient is happy, this should be no cause for concern.

On the other hand, if your patient has not been written for a premed and is suffering from pain, nausea or extreme anxiety, do not be afraid to contact the anaesthetist concerned. The symptoms may have developed since the preop visit, and you will be doing him/her a favour by alerting them to the problem.

Another problem with premeds is timing. A number of different systems operate. Premeds are sometimes written for a specific time, but this requires a considerable amount of guesswork as to the duration of the preceding operations. In some centres, the anaesthetist calls the ward when he wants the next premed given. Even this is unreliable, because it is usually at exactly this point that the surgeon realizes he left his mobile phone in the preceding patient's abdomen, or some other delaying event occurs. That many patients arrive for surgery before or after the effect of their premed is a fact of life and no-one should lose sleep over it.

The main indications for a premed are as follows:

1. *Anxiolysis.* This is the commonest indication. Anxiety is unpleasant, and in some patients, all co-operation can be lost. The most suitable anxiolytics are the benzodiazepines (e.g. diazepam 5–10 mg 1 h preop). Temazepam 10 mg is often prescribed as a shorter acting mild sedative, but it has only weak anxiolytic action.
2. *Analgesia.* Pre-existing pain should be treated as well as possible preoperatively, and an analgesic premed is a suitable way of achieving this.
3. *Drying of secretions.* An anticholinergic agent such as atropine, glyco-pyrrolate or hyoscine may be given to dry pharyngeal secretions.
4. *Alteration of stomach contents.* Premeds are often written for patients who are at special risk of aspiration in the perioperative period. Such patients include:
   - pregnant women (>16 weeks gestation);
   - those with hiatus hernia or symptoms of reflux;
   - gross obesity;
   - emergency/trauma patients.

   Medication is aimed at reducing the volume and pH of gastric contents, for example ranitidine, to prevent production of acid (50 mg i.v. or 150 mg orally) or sodium citrate, an antacid, to neutralize acid already secreted (usually 30 ml). Notice that the particulate antacids like mist. magnesium trisillicate are not used, as they cause a pneumonitis, and aspirating mist. mag. trisill. is almost as bad as inhaling acid.
5. *Other specific medications.*
   - *Hypotensive anaesthesia* – a popular technique of hypotensive anaesthesia (e.g. for middle ear surgery) involves giving a β-blocker such as atenolol 50 mg p.o. as a premed.
   - *Asthma* – it is traditional to give a dose of inhaler on leaving the ward.
   - *Angina* – some anaesthetists write for a dose of GTN, or a GTN patch to be given preop.

Starvation

Most people know that a period of fasting is required before general anaesthesia. There is, however, a great deal of confusion surrounding precise recommendations, and the reasoning behind them.

Traditional practice

The traditional order for preoperative patients is 'nil by mouth after midnight'. There are a number of problems with this approach:

- *Fluid balance* – for most patients, this means that the last oral fluid was at about 7 p.m. If the patient is not operated on until 12 noon the next day, this represents a considerable fluid deficit. This is unpleasant, and can be hazardous.
- *Medication* – many patients (and health care workers) mistakenly believe that oral medications should not be taken when nil by mouth before surgery. Withholding medication can have adverse effects.
- *Children* – HATE fasting and fluid restriction. They are even more susceptible to the fluid deficits, and smaller children may actually become hypoglycaemic after relatively short fasts.

- *Stomach pH* – there is mounting evidence that absolute starvation may in fact delay stomach emptying, and lower the pH of gastric fluid. The severity of acid-aspiration pneumonitis is closely related to the pH of the aspirate.

Current thinking

To the best of current knowledge, the following regimen is appropriate for healthy elective patients without special risks:

- Avoid solids for 4 h preop
- Clear fluids up until 2 h preop
- Oral medication taken with a sip of water **does not** increase risk
- Light, early breakfast is safe in patients on an afternoon list

It is important that patients understand that sweets and chewing gum count as solid food, and that tea and coffee are not clear fluids.

Emergencies or trauma cases. Cases may proceed without starvation if the risk of delay outweighs the risk of aspiration (e.g. cases involving haemorrhage). In all other cases, the patient should be fasted in the normal way. There is no safe and reliable alternative to a period of fasting. Metoclopramide, nasogastric suction and emetic drugs will not provide acceptable protection.

Local or regional anaesthesia. Cases booked for local or regional anaesthesia should all be starved in the normal way. This is because any local technique can fail, and general anaesthesia may become necessary. Also, most regional techniques (including Bier's block) carry potential complications, for which intubation may become necessary.

The bottom line

The biggest problem of all is logistics. Whereas it may be perfectly good science to give clear fluids up until 2 h before surgery, it's not much use if you don't know when surgery will take place (see 'premeds' above). Also, some of our patients may confuse the instructions, and eat huge greasy breakfasts before day-case surgery.

So, we're back to nil by mouth after midnight.

Regular medication

The essence of the perioperative care of patients with chronic illnesses is to get them as well as they can be before surgery, and keep them as such. It makes little sense, therefore, to bring in a beautifully controlled hypertensive and stop all his medication on the day of surgery. Be aware that:

- Very few drugs 'interfere' with anaesthesia.
- Taking pills before surgery does not increase the risk of aspiration.
- Stopping some medications, particularly for asthma, hypertension, angina or dysrhythmias, can be dangerous.

There are of course, exceptions. There are drugs which should be stopped, and many more which should cause the anaesthetist to alter his or her technique. Confusion sometimes arises about the following:

- Insulin and oral hypoglycaemics. Because of perioperative fasting, the management of diabetic therapy is inevitably altered during surgery. Hypoglycaemia under anaesthesia is dangerous and difficult to spot, so all long-acting agents are usually stopped. Beware chlorpropamide with its 36-h half-life. The perioperative care of the diabetic is covered in *exhaustive, depressing* detail in Chapter I.7.

- Antibiotics. No concern. Aminoglycosides (e.g. gentamicin) can affect the action of muscle relaxants, but the indication for the antibiotic usually outweighs this.
- Anticoagulant therapy. Clotting times usually need to be restored to normal to avoid excessive intraoperative bleeding, but it depends on the surgery and the indication for anticoagulation.
- Anticonvulsants. Should be continued. Sudden cessation can lead to severe rebound convulsions.
- Antidysrhythmics. Continue.
- Cytotoxic chemotherapy. A previous history of bleomycin therapy should always be sought in patients who have had chemotherapy. This drug may lead to severe respiratory problems, especially if given with high concentrations of oxygen. Other cytotoxic drugs are of no concern.
- Antiparkinsonian treatment. Should always be continued, to avoid rigidity and immobility postoperatively.
- Antihypertensive therapy. Continue. Rebound hypertension and cardiovascular complications are a risk if stopped, especially with older therapies such as clonidine.
- β-Blockers. Definitely continue. Cessation leads to increased incidence of myocardial ischaemia.
- Corticosteroids. Steroids should never be stopped abruptly, especially in times of stress. Patients who have been on steroids up to 1 year before surgery may have impaired stress responses, and it is traditional to give steroids in the perioperative period, parenterally if necessary. The equivalent dose of hydrocortisone i.v. is approximately four times the dose of oral prednisolone.
- Lithium. It is recommended that lithium be stopped 48–72 h before surgery. This is mainly because surgery may precipitate acute lithium toxicity as a result of alterations in renal function, and salt/water homeostasis. Lithium toxicity causes nausea, diarrhoea, weakness, tremor, slurred speech, confusion, coma and convulsions. Serum levels may be measured, toxicity being suggested by a level >2 mmol/l. It is treated with vigorous infusion of 0.9% saline.

  Lithium should be restarted as soon as possible after surgery provided renal function and fluid and electrolyte balance are normal. Acute mania is unlikely to return in this time.

- Monoamine oxidase inhibitors. Drugs in this group include phenelzine and tranylcypromine. They are used for the treatment of depression where other agents have failed. Although there are important drug interactions, it is usually recommended that MAOIs be continued.

  These agents are only now used in severe depression, and cessation carries a significant risk of suicide. Also, even with 2 weeks of cessation, interactions may occur. **Never** discontinue MAOIs without psychiatric advice.

  The following drugs must be avoided *at all costs* in those on MAOIs:

  Pethidine, fentanyl and phenoperidine. Morphine is safe.

  Dextromethorphan, which is found in 'Actifed' and 'Lotussin' cough linctuses.

Indirect-acting sympathomimetics (e.g. ephedrine or amphetamine). Interactions can cause either a hypertensive crisis, or have depressant effects. Either way, the phenomenon can be highly dangerous.

- Antipsychotic drugs. Continue, to prevent relapsing. Most (e.g. chlorpromazine) may be given i.m. Beware additive effects of other antidopaminergic drugs such as metoclopramide and prochlorperazine.
- Other antidepressants. Continue.

Drug allergies

The public perception of what comprises a true allergy is suspect, to say the least. Some patients believe they are allergic to a drug if it doesn't work.

When a patient claims to have a drug allergy, *always* ask what happened when they took it. Any history of rashes, swelling or severe illness should, of course, be taken seriously. True allergies are common to penicillins, iodine preparations and Elastoplast. Cross-sensitivity may occur to other drugs (e.g. an estimated 8% of those allergic to penicillin will react to cephalosporins).

Many other 'allergies' may not be immune reactions, but important nevertheless, for example suxamethonium apnoea, or severe dystonia after a small dose of an antiemetic. Others represent known side-effects, such as diarrhoea with antibiotics, or nausea after morphine. You can imagine what perioperative problems will be caused to a patient who claims to be allergic to morphine. Idiosyncratic reactions may also occur, and should be recorded.

Teeth and other prostheses

As a rule, anything detachable should be removed from the patient before he or she leaves the ward.

False teeth. There is a theoretical danger of loose dentures being dislodged, and either being swallowed or aspirated during surgery. They also run the risk of being lost if taken out anywhere but at the patient's bedside. For these reasons, false teeth are usually removed. However, in some centres the need for this is being re-appraised. The incidence of problems arising from well-fitting full dentures is very small, and their removal leaves an edentulous collapsing face that is difficult to mask ventilate.

A survey of patients at a major teaching hospital revealed that the thing the patients hated most of all, more than the pain, suffering, anxiety and indignity of surgery, was having to take out their teeth. Whether or not to remove teeth is therefore a matter for individual hospital policy.

Contact lenses. If these are left in they can cause corneal abrasions. They can also get lost.

Hearing aids. These are an exception. Leave them in to facilitate communication.

Jewellery. Metal jewellery can lead to diathermy burns if left exposed. Necklaces and bracelets should always be removed. Wedding rings and ear studs are OK to be left in if they are covered with tape. Any underwear with metal fasteners should also be removed for the same reason. Don't forget that, increasingly, people are having other intimate body parts pierced, and *all* rings need to be covered.

Do you know how diathermy works?

The diathermy machine passes an AC electric current through the patient. The current enters the body via the diathermy forceps and, because the contact area is small, the *current density* is high, and a burn occurs. The current then exits the body via the large grounding plate which nurses stick to the patient's leg. Here the current density is low, so no burn occurs. If the grounding plate becomes disconnected, the diathermy machine makes a noise like an air-raid siren, and switches itself off. If the patient is connected to earth by a small metal object such as a ring or bra strap, there is a risk that the current will leave the body at this point, causing an unwanted skin burn.

Nail varnish. This ought to be removed with acetone as it tends to interfere with pulse oximetry readings. Lipstick can make it hard to detect cyanosis.

False limbs, hairpieces, etc. These are not exactly hazardous, though I can remember when a toupée got in the way of an intubation once. For dignity's sake, those with wigs should probably be allowed to keep them on.

Bowel prep

This is one of medical science's more imaginative tortures. Cleansing the bowel of faecal residue is required prior to colonic surgery, colonoscopy or barium enema. Older, more protracted techniques have now largely been superseded by the use of polyethylene glycol preparations such as Klean-Prep™, Golytely™, E-Z-Dumpp™ or Plop-Be-Gone™. Actually, I made up the last two. A sachet is dissolved in 4 litres of water, and the patient drinks the lot, over a couple of hours. The first torrent will appear after about an hour.
    Bowel prep can cause abdominal pain and nausea, and may cause a significant fluid deficit. (If you don't believe me, weigh the patient before and after.) It is contraindicated in any kind of acute abdomen, in patients with impaired consciousness and in anyone weighing less than 20 kg.

Shaving

Shaving of the operative site is normally advised to reduce the incidence of wound infection. It should only be undertaken immediately before surgery, preferably after induction of anaesthesia. It has been shown that shaving the day before actually *increases* wound infection.

Deep vein thrombosis prophylaxis

Do *not* forget it. See Chapter II.23.

Antibiotic prophylaxis

Don't expect anyone to remember to give the antibiotics if you forget to write them up. There are two indications:

1. *To reduce the incidence of postoperative wound infection.* Prophylactic antibiotics given at the time of surgery are known to substantially reduce the incidence of wound infection. Two to three doses of the flavour of the month, given over 8–16 h, are enough to provide adequate prophylaxis. The precise drugs used will vary, depending on the individual firm or hospital, and factors such as cost, toxicity and efficacy are taken into account. You are unlikely to need this book to tell you what your consultant prefers, but the following is a guide:
   - biliary surgery: cephalosporin or Augmentin
   - colorectal surgery: cephalosporin with metronidazole
   - vascular surgery: cephalosporin or Augmentin
   - amputation: benzyl penicillin, metronidazole and cephalosporin
   - orthopaedics: cephalosporin

2. *To prevent endocarditis in susceptible individuals.* Those at risk are:
   - High risk: patients with prosthetic heart valves or a history of bacterial endocarditis.
   - Moderate risk: patients with rheumatic heart disease, septal defects, patent ductus, mitral valve prolapse, aortic sclerosis, a history of rheumatic fever and i.v. drug abusers.

Prophylaxis is recommended for the following procedures:
- Dental surgery
- Respiratory tract surgery
- Genitourinary procedures
- Gastrointestinal surgery ('high risk' group only).

For the vast majority of patients, the following is quite suitable:
- Amoxycillin 3 g orally 1 h preoperatively, or 1 g i.v. on induction, followed by 500 mg orally 6 h later.

If the patient is allergic to penicillin, or has taken penicillin within the last month, give:
- Clindamicin 300 mg orally 1 h preoperatively, followed by 150 mg 6 h later.

When in doubt about any high-risk case, contact your microbiologist.

Children

Children undergoing simple elective surgery are rarely under the care of paediatricians. The usual principles of perioperative management apply, but there are special considerations:
- *Fitness for surgery*: the most likely reason for postponement is an active upper respiratory tract infection. It is sometimes difficult to judge, especially with ENT cases who are always a bit snotty. However, fever, anorexia, productive cough or chest signs are definite reasons to postpone.
- *Needles*: avoid intramuscular injections if at all possible. EMLA cream should be applied at least an hour before intravenous cannulation. Preoperative blood tests are very rarely indicated in elective surgery.
- *Starvation*: more hazardous in small children. Clear fluids are safe up to

2 h preoperatively, if in a supervised environment.

- *Waiting*: children hate it. Put them first on the list if possible.
- *Parents*: can accompany their child to the anaesthetic room in most civilized hospitals, though they should not be coerced. Their job is to act as an anxiolytic, and, in most cases, they achieve this more effectively than premedication would. Anaesthesia is not a spectator sport, so one parent is enough. A minority of parents are so anxious themselves, that they make things worse, and may be excluded at the discretion of the anaesthetist. Near disasters have occurred when parents have tried to physically 'protect' an apnoeic child from the anaesthetist.
- *Clothes*: taking them from a child can cause great distress, and many children refuse to undress as a means of exerting some control over the situation. It is rarely essential to completely undress a child as you would for an adult. Keep an open mind.
- *Communications*: do everything you can think of not to appear frightening (wash that blood off your shoes), take your coat off, get down to the child's level, bring your language down too. Use a parent as a translator, but do talk to the child directly. Don't chase the poor little things around the ward, go on talking to the parents and most children will come to find out what's going on. Whatever else you do, get the trust of the parents. If they are unhappy they will transmit it to the child.
- *Honesty*: some children are admitted for elective surgery, having been told by their parents that they are going to the library. If you lie to children, they won't trust you. Generally speaking, the more honest you are about needles, etc., the better.

Chapter I.4

EMERGENCIES

Chapter I.4

EMERGENCIES

KEY POINTS

Urgency determines timing of surgery.
Any acutely ill patient needs resuscitation along the lines of ABCDE.
For any acute admission, consider fluids, analgesia, oxygen, naso-
gastric tube, urinary catheter and deep vein thrombosis prophylaxis.

Estimating urgency

In the good old days, operations were carried out around the clock by the
registrar rather than interfere with the consultant's golfing schedule. Recently,
the Royal Colleges of Surgeons and of Anaesthetists realized that having
surgery performed at 4 a.m. by a sleep-deprived junior was less than ideal,
and commissioned NCEPOD (the National Confidential Enquiry into Peri-
Operative Deaths). This was important because it proved that surgery should
be performed by staff of adequate seniority and experience, and at a sensible
time of day.

NCEPOD categorizes cases in terms of urgency into four bands:

1. *Elective.* No risk to the patient is caused by delay, therefore surgery
   proceeds only when any other medical problems are optimally
   controlled. These cases are done only in normal working hours. Note that
   some elective cases still require careful timing to bring them to theatre in
   peak condition (e.g. control of thyrotoxicosis before thyroidectomy).
2. *Scheduled.* These cases need to proceed within a period of 2–3 weeks
   because of actual or potential worsening of the surgical pathology
   (typically malignancies). There is time to control most medical problems,
   but it may be unavoidable to incur some extra risk (e.g. operation within
   3 months of an MI). These cases belong in normal working hours.
3. *Urgent.* The surgical pathology demands operation within 24 h. This
   category includes the majority of the patients admitted 'on take' (e.g.
   fractures, drainage of abscesses, appendicectomy, etc.). Surgery proceeds
   after resuscitation and is frequently performed out of hours. However,
   operating after midnight should be avoided unless there is a threat to life
   or limb. Ideally, an emergency theatre is kept open during the day to
   lessen the load at night.
4. *Emergency.* Sometimes surgery is part of the resuscitation (usually in the
   control of major haemorrhage); these patients are much too sick *not* to
   have an operation. These cases proceed immediately, day or night, and
   less urgent cases have to make way for them, however inconvenient this
   may be.

Thus there is a *window of opportunity* for every case. The correct time to operate is judged by balancing the risk of delay against the risk of going ahead, for example:

- Appendicitis, unwell for 3 days with lots of vomiting. Benefits from a few hours delay for rehydration and correction of hypokalaemia.
- Perforated duodenal ulcer. Peritonitis with worsening shock will progress rapidly after perforation. You have 1–2 h to resuscitate and only partial correction of acidosis and electrolyte disturbance may be possible.
- Ruptured aortic aneurysm, rapidly worsening hypotension and acidosis. The surgery *is* the resuscitation. Proceed immediately.

Priorities in resuscitation in trauma

The severely injured patient needs a slightly different approach from the exhaustive and methodical history–exam–investigation system that serves so well for elective cases. Firstly, treatment and assessment are conducted **in tandem.** Secondly, assessment is **prioritized** so that the most immediately life-threatening problems are dealt with before moving on to lesser threats. When faced with a really ill patient, think **ABCDE** and you will be able to start resuscitation instead of collapsing in a gibbering panic. Also, be sure to pack extra underwear when on take.

A *is for airway.* Nothing kills quicker than asphyxia. For rapid evaluation get the patient to talk to you. Any stridor, tracheal tug or intercostal recession indicates obstruction. Simple measures to relieve this are: to clear the mouth with a gloved finger; to use suction; to open the mouth and lift the jaw forward; to insert an oral airway; to insert a nasal airway. The trauma patient must be assumed to have a broken neck and you must protect the cervical spine while clearing the airway. In-line manual stabilization is very effective. These manual airway skills are not easily learnt from a book; the best way is to practice on live anaesthetized patients in theatre. It need only take a few minutes to learn a life-saving technique.

Obstruction, coma, deep neck wounds and facial burns are indications for urgent and expert airway control. Call an anaesthetist. It is better to put out a crash-call before actual arrest to ensure that you get a quick response. Amateur intubations are only justified if the patient arrests and an expert is not available. Under no circumstances should you ever use paralysing drugs; the arrested patient doesn't need them, anyone else is likely to be killed by them.

Only after sorting out the airway can you move on to the next stage.

B *is for breathing.* Trauma patients may have pneumothoraces (simple or tension), open chest wounds or haemothoraces. All of these are life-threatening and will be missed unless you have a high level of suspicion and actively look for them. The principal signs are respiratory rate, tracheal deviation and auscultated breath sounds.

All trauma cases will benefit from an oxygen mask with a reservoir (yes, even those with COAD). Now you may proceed to C.

C *is for circulation.* See also Chapter II.7. Assess pulse rate, skin colour, mental state, blood pressure and urine output. Establish large-bore i.v. access and send bloods at the same time (FBC, electrolytes, clotting and cross-match). Start generous fluid resuscitation (with a salt solution) and reassess frequently for a return to normal urine output and blood pressure.

D is for (neurological) disability. You need not lose time on a full examination. The important facts are given by the level of consciousness and by the pupil size and reactivity. Inequality of the pupils may indicate an expanding intracranial lesion. A low level of consciousness is a non-specific sign, but any changes are important as an early indicator of worsening shock or of raised intracranial pressure. This is best quantified by the Glasgow Coma Scale (GCS).

The Glasgow Coma Scale		Score
Eye-opening	spontaneous	4
	in response to speech	3
	in response to pain	2
	none	1
Verbal response	normal, orientated	5
	confused	4
	inappropriate words	3
	noises, no words	2
	none	1
Best motor response	obeys commands	6
	purposeful pain response	5
	withdraws from pain	4
	abnormal flexion to pain	3
	abnormal extension to pain	2
	none	1

The best possible score is 15. A GCS of 3 is what you get for turning up.

E is for exposure. In all cases, but especially in trauma, it is necessary to undress the patient or pathologies will go undetected. Ill patients are at high risk of hypothermia, so you must cover them with warm blankets.

If you follow these headings you will make considerable progress towards resuscitation within the first few minutes of the admission, but most importantly you will prevent unnecessary deaths. Following this scheme should also allow you to keep your head when the severity of the case appears overwhelming.

Head injury

The patient with a severe head injury clearly requires expert management from a neurosurgeon and will usually be referred to ITU. However, as a house surgeon, you will frequently have to deal with patients with less severe injury who also need surgery (typically as the result of assaults or road accidents). Success depends upon identifying the presence of head injury, the presence of associated injuries and early detection of any changes. Following a thorough examination, radiological tests are central to the diagnosis.

Cervical spine X-ray. A high quality lateral view of the cervical spine is indicated for all patients with head injury. Leave a cervical collar in place until the films have been reviewed by someone of adequate experience.

Skull X-ray. Any suspicion of skull penetration or depression, deep lacerations, extensive bruises, CSF leakage or evidence of a skull base fracture (two black eyes or bruising over the mastoid process) should lead to a skull X-ray. All cases with a history of unconsciousness or with any abnormal neurology should also be X-rayed.

CT scanning. All patients with a skull fracture, with a GCS <8 or with abnormal signs need a CT scan. Any patient whose GCS falls by two points needs an urgent repeat scan. Headaches or confusion lasting into the second day after injury also need repeat scans. Ideally, all patients who need anaesthesia following an episode of unconsciousness should be scanned first.

Managing head injury

1. *Observations*. Put the patient in an area where they are easy to observe. Repeat GCS measurements at hourly intervals. Measure vital signs frequently (at least every 4 h, depending on the overall situation). Include an assessment of pupil size, equality and reactivity in the charting.
2. *Analgesia*. While it is true that over-sedation is potentially harmful, these patients should not be denied analgesia. Pain may be detrimental to the injured brain because of swings in blood pressure and because of hypoxia (e.g. from fractured ribs inhibiting respiration). The safest way to achieve analgesia is with titration of small i.v. doses of opioid (e.g. with a patient-controlled analgesia pump – see Chapter II.4) followed by frequent reassessments.
3. *Oxygen*. A face mask is compulsory for all these cases. The injured brain is exquisitely sensitive to hypoxia.
4. *Fluids*. Fluid therapy appropriate to the patient's injuries and surgery must be continued despite the head injury. Overzealous use of large amounts of crystalloids may precipitate cerebral oedema, but the much greater risk is that of hypovolaemia. The injured brain doesn't tolerate hypotension and reduced perfusion. In practice, it is safe to give a reduced maintenance dose of fluid (typically 2 l per day) and be prepared to use colloids in boluses to treat oliguria or tachycardia. An increased level of monitoring is needed.
5. *Other drugs*. Antibiotics or anticonvulsants may be indicated where there is evidence of fracture; consult the regional neurosurgery unit.

What not to do to head injuries

Never assume that a reduced level of consciousness is due to alcohol.
Never allow a head injured patient to remain hypotensive or hypoxic.
Never send a semi-conscious patient to an area where the level of observation is low (e.g. X-ray) without an appropriate escort.
Never transfer a patient by ambulance without an appropriate escort and level of airway protection (ask for advice from an anaesthetist).

Resuscitation for surgical patients

Virtually all surgical emergencies can be predicted to suffer pain and dehydration. Many will also have bleeding or biochemical disturbance.

- **Fluids:** it is never wrong to put up a drip, though it is not always necessary. It is important to replace large fluid deficits, see Chapter II.6 for details.
- **Analgesia:** it is reasonable to withhold analgesia until an appropriate assessment is made. This means that surgical assessment needs to be made promptly. Once a diagnosis has been made, or particularly if the decision to operate has been reached, there is no excuse for not providing adequate analgesia. See Chapters II.1–II.4.
- **Oxygen:** any patient who is remotely sick requires oxygen.
- **Equipment:** consider venous access, urinary catheter, nasogastric tube.
- **DVT prophylaxis:** start it immediately where not contraindicated (e.g. minihep and stockings).

Chapter I.5

PRE-EXISTING CARDIOVASCULAR DISEASE

Chapter I.5

Pre-existing Cardiovascular Disease

Key Points

The usual principle applies: optimize the treatment of any medical condition before surgery. This is especially important with hypertension and heart disease.

Do not hesitate to contact the physicians if you feel improvement can be made, but do not ask them whether the patient is 'fit for anaesthetic'.

Introduction

For any form of cardiovascular disease that is poorly controlled, optimization of therapy by the medical team will improve overall morbidity and mortality. If you can predict such problems in advance, you may save your patient avoidable delays.

A physician's expertise lies in judging whether or not the patient's medical disorder is optimally treated. Please do not ask physicians to give opinions on 'fitness for anaesthetic', even if this sometimes amounts to the same thing. It never ceases to astound me that some cardiologists feel they should write 'fit for a light GA' in the notes, and I usually invite them to come and give this intriguing form of anaesthesia themselves.

Hypertension

Hypertension is common amongst surgical patients. Most patients are on appropriate treatment, but a significant number may be poorly controlled or may present for the first time when admitted for surgery. Adequate treatment of pre-existing hypertension reduces mortality and morbidity in the perioperative period.

Uncontrolled hypertensives subjected to surgery tend to exhibit grossly exaggerated blood pressure responses (both up and down) to surgical and anaesthetic stimuli. These swings persist after surgery and are implicated in the development of strokes and myocardial infarction.

The cut-off for the definition of 'poorly controlled hypertension' is **diastolic of 110 mmHg**. There are three situations you may face:

1. *Well controlled hypertensives.* No readings above 110 mmHg diastolic. Routine preparation of the hypertensive should include the following:
   - Maintain all antihypertensive medication throughout the perioperative period, wherever possible.
   - Preoperative investigations should involve an ECG. Evidence of left

ventricular hypertrophy or 'strain' suggests higher risk. U&Es are indicated if the patient is on diuretics.
- Bear in mind that hypertension is associated with ischaemic heart disease, and such patients should receive 'MI prophylaxis' measures (see Chapter II.14)

2. *Poorly controlled hypertension, elective surgery.* This may take many forms:
   - Severe undiagnosed hypertension with persistent diastolic elevation should be investigated and treated before surgery. This usually means sending the patient back to the GP and re-admitting after a month or so.
   - Borderline hypertension (e.g. one reading above 110 mmHg), in someone who is already on treatment, is more difficult. It is not uncommon to send such patients home to their GPs, who find that their blood pressure is perfectly normal. Such 'White coat hypertension' is probably not a risk, but the anaesthetist should be contacted if in doubt.

3. *Urgent surgery in poorly controlled hypertensives.* The management of acute hypertension is more difficult still. The risk posed by surgery is probably reduced by acute therapy, but rapid reduction of blood pressure can, of itself, be dangerous, especially in the elderly. Such patients should always be referred to the medical team if urgent therapy is considered.

Cardiac failure

Patients with cardiac failure form a wide spectrum. The patient with end-stage disease is easy to recognize and presents a very high risk for any kind of surgery. Lesser degrees of failure may be harder to spot, and assessing risk of surgery may be difficult. Features to look for are:

1. *History.* Exercise tolerance is a sensitive measure of cardiac reserve and fitness for surgery. A patient who can walk a mile on the flat or climb a flight of stairs is likely to tolerate anaesthesia. Worry about patients who get breathless chewing their food. Past history of myocardial infarctions or other hospital admissions, and cardiac medication should be sought. Orthopnoea and paroxysmal nocturnal dyspnoea should be documented.

2. *Examination.* Any sign of overt failure should send you scurrying to phone a physician, and the earlier the better. Tachycardia at rest, severe lower limb oedema, raised JVP, gallop rhythm, basal crepitations. Murmurs should be noted, but *new* murmurs need a cardiologist's evaluation before surgery.

3. *Investigations.*
   - ECG is mandatory before surgery of any kind. Look for dysrhythmias, old MI and acute ischaemia.
   - An echocardiogram arguably gives more information about fitness of the heart to tolerate anaesthesia and surgery than any other test. It can demonstrate valve lesions and estimate gradients as a guide to severity. It can look at motility of the myocardium, which may detect old MI or ongoing ischaemia. Most important of all, it can give an accurate assessment of **ejection fraction**, which is the best predictor of outcome for major surgery. An ejection fraction of <40% should provoke a serious re-think as to the wisdom of any big operation. Consider requesting an echo for anyone with new murmurs or severe

exercise limitation, especially in patients requiring major surgery (e.g. aortic aneurysm repair).

Patients with poor left ventricular function may still require surgery, and, if so, a postoperative intensive care unit bed should be arranged. Occasionally, it may be appropriate for cardiac surgery to be carried out before the planned procedure.

- Other tests (e.g. exercise tolerance test, angiography, MUGA scans, etc.) are not usually done unless recommended by a cardiologist. A chest X-ray may be justified, especially if not done in the preceding year. A full blood count should be done and a lower than usual threshold for treating anaemia adopted. U&E is indicated, especially if the patient is on diuretics.

Patients with heart failure often pose fluid balance problems, but unnecessarily so (see Chapter II.6).

Valvular heart disease

Severe valve disease is becoming less common, but still presents in the surgical ward from time to time. The preoperative management is as for cardiac failure, and those with good exercise tolerance are unlikely to cause trouble. Patients to spot are those with *fixed cardiac output states*, that is aortic stenosis, mitral stenosis, constrictive pericarditis. These patients react badly to vasodilation, and cardiovascular collapse is not uncommon on induction of anaesthesia if the problem is not detected. It is not unreasonable to request further evaluation (i.e. echocardiogram) for any patient with:

- a new murmur (developed during the course of the acute illness);
- known aortic stenosis;
- long-standing murmurs associated with poor exercise tolerance.

Occasionally, cardiac surgery to replace the diseased valve is indicated prior to elective surgery.

Patients with *prosthetic heart valves* rarely cause haemodynamic problems, but need heavy anticoagulation at all times. This can cause problems in the perioperative period, depending on the type of surgery. Warfarin is usually replaced by heparin, which may take several days to achieve. Patients with prosthetic valves are at high risk of developing endocarditis and require antibiotic cover (see Chapter I.3).

Ischaemic heart disease

Ischaemic heart disease is the most prolific perioperative killer. Silent ischaemia is common, occurring in up to 2.5% of the population aged 40–60. Perioperative management of ischaemic heart disease is covered in Chapter II.14.

Situations that should ring particular preoperative alarm bells are:

1. *Recent myocardial infarction.* It is rarely in the patient's interest to perform elective, non-cancer surgery within 6 months of a myocardial infarction.
2. *'Unstable angina'.* Angina which has recently changed in frequency or severity, or in which the effort required to produce chest pain has reduced significantly, carries a much higher perioperative risk. Increased GTN consumption is a sensitive measure of this. Such patients should be referred to a cardiologist for assessment and management.

Dysrhythmias

Patients treated for dysrhythmias require the same assessment as any other cardiac patient. The most common abnormality is atrial fibrillation (AF). Points to remember are:

- Ventricular rate in controlled AF should be about 80 b.p.m. Question the adequacy of treatment if it is higher.
- Maintain all antidysrhythmics throughout the perioperative period. Contact a cardiologist for advice if parenteral therapy is likely to be necessary.
- Beware hypokalaemia or changes in renal function in patients on digoxin. If digoxin levels are thought necessary, blood should be taken 6 h after the dose is given. Random digoxin levels are useless.

Other stuff

Congenital heart disease

This can range from a simple, asymptomatic septal defect, to severe cyanotic heart disease. The most important thing to remember for all of them is antibiotic prophylaxis (see Chapter II.3). If difficulties arise, particularly in urgent surgery, contact the cardiologist involved in the case. Note that, even for the adults, this will often be a *paediatric* cardiologist.

Hypertrophic obstructive cardiomyopathy (HOCM)

This is a congenital condition which causes eccentric hypertrophy of the cardiac septum, leading to both impaired filling, and outflow obstruction. Dysrhythmias are common and may be fatal. A cardiological assessment is always a good idea prior to anaesthesia.

Problems in the perioperative period may occur if tachycardia or hypovolaemia are allowed to develop. Vasodilators should be avoided. Close monitoring (e.g. on a high dependency unit or CCU) is valuable.

Wolff–Parkinson–White syndrome

This is a congenital abnormality of the conducting system. An accessory pathway (the bundle of Kent) connects atria and ventricles. Patients are at risk of paroxysmal re-entrant tachycardia (see Chapter II.12), and may be on medication. ECG shows a short P–R interval (usually <0.12 sec) best seen in lead V1, and a delta wave before the QRS complex. Tachydysrythmias in affected individuals should be treated with physiological manoeuvres first, for example Valsalva, carotid sinus massage.

Pacemakers

The insertion of a permanent transvenous pacemaker is an effective and cost-effective way of treating symptomatic heart block, both paroxysmal and permanent. Patients with pacemakers frequently present for surgery, and may be anxious about the functioning of the device during anaesthesia and surgery. Patients with pacemakers have heart disease and as such need to be handled carefully, but there are no special precautions for pacemaker patients. Although there is a theoretical danger of reprogramming of the device when exposed to diathermy current, the incidence of problems is very low.

Chapter I.6

PRE-EXISTING RESPIRATORY DISEASE

Chapter I.6

PRE-EXISTING RESPIRATORY DISEASE

Smoking

Smoking and surgery do not mix. Apart from the long-term effects on
cardiorespiratory health, smoking makes airways irritable, increases sputum
production, impairs ciliary function, reduces immunity, increases vascular
resistance, increases risk of deep vein thrombosis and reduces oxygen delivery
by carbon monoxide poisoning. Postoperative chest infection is six times more
likely in smokers after abdominal surgery compared with non-smokers.
Smoking may also impair wound healing, especially in plastic surgery.

Effects of stopping smoking

Chronic smokers can improve their surgical outcome if they quit 4–6
weeks before surgery, and should be encouraged to do so. Stopping for...

12–24 h	benefits the cardiovascular system by reducing the need for carbon monoxide and nicotine elimination.
3–4 days	improves ciliary activity.
1–2 weeks	reduces sputum volume.
6 weeks	reduces pulmonary and coronary vascular resistance, restores normal pulmonary macrophage function.

Fitness for surgery

Notice this section is not entitled 'fitness for anaesthesia'. The most
important determinant of outcome in a respiratory patient is the nature of
surgery. As always, the determination of fitness for a particular operation is
based on a risk–benefit assessment, which in difficult cases is made jointly
between surgeon and anaesthetist.

The first consideration, as ever, is whether the patient is a fit as he can be.

It is essential to exclude intercurrent chest infection in chronic chest disease. When in doubt, ask the opinion of a chest physician, who can give advice about optimal treatment for the perioperative period.

Obese chest patients should be encouraged to lose weight. Malnourished chest patients may benefit from a period of artificial feeding preoperatively. All patients should be encouraged to give up smoking.

Local or regional anaesthesia can avoid problems for some forms of surgery, but remember that some patients are too sick to be operated on *without* a general anaesthetic. For example, a patient who cannot stop coughing or lie flat is not suitable for cataract extraction under local anaesthesia.

Asthma

Most patients with asthma have mild disease which is well controlled. The occasional patient with poorly controlled asthma is difficult to anaesthetize, and advanced warning will be appreciated by the anaesthetist. Most severe asthmatics see a chest physician regularly, and his/her help should be sought early in the piece, to ensure appropriate perioperative management.

- To gauge the severity of asthma, ask about previous admissions, courses of steroids, admissions to the intensive care unit, and limitation of activities. Severe asthmatics are rarely wheeze-free.
- Maintain *all* regular medication throughout the postoperative period, using parenteral preparations if necessary. Enlist the help of a physician for complex drug regimens, especially where theophylline derivatives have been prescribed.
- For severe asthma, respiratory function tests may be appropriate, and may help a physician in his assessment. For well-controlled asthma, extra tests (e.g. chest X-ray) are not normally required.
- Avoid using drugs associated with bronchospasm: morphine, diamorphine, papaveretum (pethidine or fentanyl are preferred), all NSAIDs and β-blockers are the most important.
- If oxygen is given by mask, humidify it. Treat pain adequately, try and avoid causing unnecessary anxiety.

Exacerbations of asthma in the perioperative period are considered in Chapter II.17.

'Others'

The 'others' category will mainly consist of chronic obstructive airways disease.

Assessment

Pay particular attention to:

History. The history is the best measure of severity. Exercise tolerance is a good measure of respiratory reserve and is the best way of distinguishing 'a bit of bronchitis' from respiratory cripple-dom. Remember that the definition of chronic bronchitis depends on a history of purulent sputum. The patient's own opinion of the state of his chest is relevant ("Not too bad at the moment, Doc"). Check current medications, and make a note if recently on steroids. Ask about use of NSAIDs, to identify those that can safely be given to that patient. Ask about prior admissions for chest disease, especially if ventilated, and other things such as home oxygen for severe disease. History of smoking should be sought.

Examination. Make note of temperature. Look for cyanosis, wheeze, dyspnoea at rest, right heart failure (as demonstrated by raised jugular venous pressure and peripheral oedema), clubbing or focal chest signs.

Investigations. Full blood count is always indicated, looking for raised white cell count (signalling possible chest infection) or polycythaemia, which may need to be treated before elective surgery. A chest X-ray can usually be justified, especially in the elderly but, if the patient's clinical condition has been stable, a recent film (up to a year old) will do.

For major surgery or severe disease, baseline arterial blood gases should be sent. For patients with a low P_aO_2 on air (e.g. <70 mmHg, 9 kPa) or a high P_aCO_2, it may be worth a trial of **controlled oxygen therapy** (see Chapter II.17) to find the highest inspired oxygen concentration that the patient will tolerate.

Pulmonary function tests should be done in severe disease, to measure vital capacity, FEV_1, and the response to bronchodilator therapy. ECG should be done in all cases.

Preparation

Much of the preparation of a bad chest patient is time-consuming, so the first thing to do is admit well in advance of major surgery, that is up to 48 h. Think of:

- General things: stop smoking, optimize nutrition.
- Sputum: 48 h intensive physiotherapy for bad sputum retainers.
- Wheeze: ensure adequate therapy, continue medication throughout the perioperative period. Send the inhalers to theatre with the patient.
- Cor pulmonale, etc.: if uncontrolled, this can lead to serious cardio-vascular instability in the perioperative period. Adequate management as recommended by physicians.
- ITU: for some high-risk patients, surgery may be conditional upon the availability of an intensive care unit bed for postoperative management. Warn the unit well in advance, and be prepared to postpone surgery if a bed is not available.
- DVT prophylaxis: as usual.
- Venesection: may be required for secondary polycythaemia. Consider where haemoglobin is greater than 15 g/dl.
- Antibiotics: some patients are on long-term antibiotics, and advice about continuation should be sought preoperatively.

Chapter I.7

PRE-EXISTING ENDOCRINOLOGY

Chapter I.7

PRE-EXISTING ENDOCRINOLOGY

KEY POINTS

Diabetics: High risk for heart, renal, infective and neurological disease
Need both glucose and insulin to avoid cells starving
Hypoglycaemia kills quickly, hyperglycaemia slowly
May become temporarily insulin dependent
Many regimes available; all depend on frequent glucose analysis.

Thyroid: Control thyrotoxicosis before surgery
Extra tests for the airway and parathyroid function
Postop risks are airway obstruction and hypocalcaemia.

Adrenal: Continue or increase steroid cover during surgery
Beware of iatrogenic diabetes.

Diabetes

Principles of management

Diabetes mellitus is a collective term for a variety of insulin deficiency states. For simplicity, they can be grouped together regardless of aetiology.

Diabetes covers a range of severity from very mild diet-controlled to severe 'brittle' insulin dependency. Patients also present for a range of surgery from minor to major and may be elective or emergency cases. Despite this variety, they share the same problems: metabolic; cardiovascular; infective; renal; neurological. Metabolic control is discussed below.

- **CVS:** all diabetics are at increased risk of MI, peripheral vascular disease and CVA. Meticulous examination is essential, backed by ECGs (even in young adults). Ischaemia is often occult.
- **Infective:** infection worsens control of diabetes; diabetics are immunocompromised. Early detection and treatment is necessary. Consider preop antibiotics. Rigid exclusion of urinary and respiratory infection is needed.
- **Renal:** diabetes causes chronic renal failure. This must be detected preop so that further deterioration can be prevented. U&Es must be measured.
- **Neurological:** a potentially deadly complication is autonomic neuropathy which can cause crashing hypotension (making MI and CVA more likely). This is detected on clinical examination by abolition of the sinus arrhythmia, abnormal response to Valsalva manoeuvre (pulse rate

does not change during forced expiration against a closed glottis) and by postural hypotension (>20 mmHg drop on standing).

Principles of metabolic control

Diabetes spoils surgery by increasing infection rates and inhibiting healing. Surgery spoils diabetic control through starvation, infection and the release of stress hormones (steroids/adrenaline and growth hormone which inhibit insulin's actions). Good control prevents this vicious circle developing.

The principle action of insulin is to regulate glucose production and its uptake in cells. Without insulin, a high plasma glucose does not guarantee cellular nutrition (the body 'starves in the midst of plenty'). Diabetics need both sugar and insulin. However, uptake into the brain, which relies almost entirely on glucose for its energy, does not depend on insulin. Therefore, hyperglycaemia affects the CNS only indirectly and slowly through acid–base and electrolyte disturbance, while hypoglycaemia leads to problems very rapidly.

Many hospitals will have their own guidelines for choosing a regime. Please follow these, as non-conformism will breed confusion and unrest. Talk to your anaesthetist, who will be thrilled to help. The choice of regime depends upon the patient and on the type of surgery.

Non-insulin-dependent (NIDDMs). For **minor elective surgery**: the emphasis is on preventing hypoglycaemia and on an early return to normal eating and medication. Put these early on the list. Starve them in the usual way. Stop long-acting hypoglycaemics (**metformin, chlorpropamide**) at least 18 h preop and stop all hypoglycaemics on the morning of surgery. Check the BM stick in the morning and again just before surgery for extra brownie-points. If hypoglycaemic (unlikely) put up a 5% dextrose infusion. If glucose is >15 mmol/l inform the anaesthetist but do not start insulin.

For **major elective surgery**: these should be expected to become insulin dependent and to need an insulin–glucose regimen (see below).

For **emergency surgery**: patients with minor emergencies are at risk of hypoglycaemia due to starvation and continued hypoglycaemics. All will need blood glucose monitoring (e.g. 4-hourly) and most will need i.v. glucose (e.g. dextrose 5% 100 ml/h). Major emergencies will need an insulin–glucose regimen.

Newly diagnosed: elective admissions with positive urinalysis for glucose should have a laboratory blood glucose analysis. Values of >10 mmol/l random or >7 mmol/l starving probably indicate diabetes. Elective cases should be postponed for a definite diagnosis. Emergencies will need insulin and glucose.

Insulin-dependent. For **minor elective surgery**: the general considerations are as for NIDDMs. Omit long-acting insulins the night before, continuing the short-acting ones with the evening meal. Omit all insulins on the morning of surgery. Feed the patient as soon as possible postoperatively and give their usual short-acting insulin. Return to normal feeding and the usual insulin regime in the evening. Monitor blood glucose 4-hourly.

For **intermediate surgery** (a return to normal diet predicted within 1–2 days): for the newly diagnosed emergency, for major cases in the previously non-insulin-dependent, and for intermediate surgery in the insulin-dependent diabetic, an insulin–glucose regimen is indicated. See 'Action plan for insulin regimens', page 272'.

For surgery where **prolonged starvation** is likely: *dextrose solutions have negligible nutritional value.* These patients need expert help from a dietician and are likely to need both intravenous feeding and an insulin infusion. Consider an ITU bed.

Worst-case scenario: severe illness (e.g. peritonitis) may precipitate both surgery and diabetic ketoacidosis (DKA). The main metabolic disturbances in DKA are *hypovolaemia, acidosis, hyponatraemia and hyperglycaemia.* Very rapid correction of all these problems is neither possible nor desirable preoperatively (it may cause other electrolyte imbalance and cerebral oedema). Start to correct the hypovolaemia with generous amounts of saline (~ 2 l/h), give a bolus of insulin (20 units Actrapid), start monitoring vital signs and urine output and *get help.* The serum potassium, which may start off at a normal value, will plummet. Begin replacements right from the start by adding 20 mmol of KCl to each litre of saline. Measure serum potassium very frequently (hourly). Continue insulin therapy (~10 units/h) while monitoring the blood glucose. As the insulin acts, the serum glucose will fall; when it reaches 10 mmol/l start glucose replacement (dextrose 10% 100 ml/h). See 'Action plan for diabetic ketoacidosis', page 266'. These cases are very difficult indeed and definitely need an ITU bed.

Other endocrine problems

Only conditions directly relevant to the house surgeon are covered here. Very rare or very complex endocrine problems are best left to the experts.

Hyperthyroidism

Patients may present for thyroid surgery or with coincidental disease. Important baseline tests before thyroid surgery are:

- Thyroid function tests. Elective cases should always be euthyroid. Surgery without control of hyperthyroidism risks a 'thyroid storm', an uncontrolled release of thyroxine. Since this is usually fatal it's worth avoiding.
- Indirect laryngoscopy. This can be arranged through the ENT department and is intended to exclude a pre-existing laryngeal nerve palsy (which is not uncommon). If the other, normal, laryngeal nerve were to be injured in surgery the resulting bilateral palsy could threaten the airway.
- CXR and thoracic inlet views, or CT scans. These are indicated to assess the risk of tracheal compression or erosion when there is a large or a retrosternal goitre.
- Calcium (taken without a tourniquet). Unintentional excision of or injury to the parathyroids may happen at thyroidectomy and may cause hypocalcaemia. Preoperative calcium is a useful baseline study.

Preoperative control of hyperthyroidism is achieved with carbimazole and/or β-blockers, which should not be withdrawn suddenly because of rebound hypertension. Lugol's iodine is sometimes given to reduce the vascularity of the gland. Postop problems of thyroidectomy include airway obstruction due to haematoma, oedema, nerve palsies or cartilage erosion. A pair of scissors or staple removers, as appropriate, must be at the bedside to allow evacuation of haematoma. For all airway problems call an anaesthetist, put out a crash call if you have to. Acute hypoparathyroidism may occur as above. Check calcium postop and be aware that in this case tetany might not be due to a panic attack. Should hypocalcaemia happen, give i.v. calcium gluconate 10% 10 ml slowly. This is likely to need repeated doses.

Hypothyroidism
The treated and stable patient counts as normal and poses no special problems. Clinically or biochemically hypothyroid patients are at risk of heart failure, hypothermia, over-sedation and chest infections. Elective cases should be postponed until adequately treated.

Adrenocortical problems
Addisonian crisis is rare but occasionally presents as an acute abdomen. These patients are hypotensive, hyponatraemic and hyperkalaemic. Resuscitation is with saline and i.v. steroids. Stable, chronic cases of Addison's are maintained on glucocorticoids (e.g. prednisolone) and mineralocorticoids (e.g. fludrocortisone). Electrolytes and glucose should be measured preoperatively. Both types of steroid should be continued through the perioperative period, and increased doses of glucocorticoid are usual (see below).

Most patients on long-term steroid therapy are using them as anti-inflammatories or as immunosuppressants. The underlying disease should usually indicate thorough investigation (e.g. rheumatoid arthritis). All patients on steroids certainly need screening for infections, diabetes and abnormal electrolytes. Do not forget that they are also at risk of ulcers and protect them accordingly. Traditionally, though with little evidence, the glucocorticoid dose is increased at the time of surgery. Hydrocortisone 100 mg is given at induction of anaesthesia and at 8-hourly intervals for the first day. After that, the dose is halved each day until the preop dose is reached; a possible side-effect is to render the patient temporarily diabetic. For those who cannot take oral drugs postop, hydrocortisone 100 mg (i.v. or i.m.) is equivalent to prednisolone 25 mg orally. Steroids must certainly not be withdrawn abruptly as this will cause circulatory collapse.

Diabetes insipidus
This form of diabetes is not common but may follow head injury or neurosurgery. It is due to a failure of the production or action of antidiuretic hormone, which results in large volumes of dilute urine (specific gravity 1.010, osmolality <279 mOsmol/kg). The conscious patient will get very thirsty and life-threatening dehydration may develop. Treatment is with intra-nasal DDAVP (a synthetic ADH) 10–40 mcg/day. Don't worry, the packaging of DDAVP includes detailed instructions.

Chapter I.8

NEUROMUSCULAR DISEASES AND SURGERY

Chapter I.8

NEUROMUSCULAR DISEASES AND SURGERY

KEY POINTS

Many neurological and myological diseases have in common the problems of weakness, slow mobilization, inability for self-care, poor nutritional status and a predisposition to infection.

There may be special considerations such as associated cardiac disease and drug interactions.

Epilepsy

Epileptic patients pose few special problems. Those who are well controlled can be regarded as normal. Some anticonvulsants can cause blood dyscrasias (carbamazepine, phenytoin, phenobarbitone and sodium valproate) and it is worth checking an FBC. Do not discontinue any anticonvulsants as there is a risk of rebound fitting. Phenothiazines (chlorpromazine, prochlorperazine) lower the fit threshold and shouldn't be used.

Strokes

Whatever the exact mechanism of a CVA, it is fair to assume that there is an underlying arteriopathy and/or cardiac disease, so all these patients need an ECG preoperatively. Multiple small infarcts are a common cause of dementia, which may lead to problems with drug compliance and communication. Acquired skeletal deformity and immobility put the patient at high risk of deep vein thrombosis and skin breakdown. Swallowing difficulty predisposes to aspiration pneumonia and to malnutrition.

Postoperatively, patients with CVA are at high risk of chest and urinary infections. Hypovolaemia and hypoxia must be avoided at all costs. Oxygen should be prescribed (see Chapter II.17) and physiotherapy is essential. Many cases will benefit from the dietician's advice.

Rarely, surgery is indicated shortly after a CVA. Ideally, any elective surgery should be delayed until the neurological symptoms are stable and an interval of 3–6 months has passed. Any antihypertensives should be continued perioperatively and the blood pressure must be closely monitored. Pathological or iatrogenic anticoagulation must be reversed temporarily.

Parkinson's disease

As well as the general problems described above, Parkinsonians may have further respiratory compromise due to rigidity of the thorax. Continue antiParkinsonian drugs, but watch for side-effects such as urinary retention and confusion. Central dopamine antagonists may worsen Parkinsonism and should be avoided (droperidol, haloperidol, metoclopramide).

Multiple sclerosis

Legend has it that surgery or anaesthesia may cause a relapse, but the evidence is weak. The risk of UTI or chest infection is high. MS sufferers may have a bulbar palsy which puts them at risk of aspiration. Severe cases, in which there is effectively a complete spinal cord disruption, may give a history of autonomic hyperreflexia. In this condition, a stimulus such as pain, a full bladder or constipation may lead to an uncontrolled autonomic reflex with severe hypertension, sweating and bradycardia. Prevention is by good catheter and bowel care.

Motor neurone disease

Severe weakness is the norm. Bulbar palsy is common and there may be apparent signs of extremes of mood, such as crying, which do not always reflect the patients true feelings.

Myotonia

Dystrophia myotonica is rare, but worth a mention because it is bad news and because if you do diagnose it on a ward round you will look unbelievably cool. The signs are an inability to loosen the grip (after a handshake), balding, ptosis, cataracts and hypogonadism. There is an important association with severe cardiomyopathy and with diabetes. The weakness gets worse with cold. Yes, since you ask, I did diagnose it on a ward round, and yes, it was unbelievably cool.

Myasthenia gravis

This autoimmune disease affecting the motor end plate is particularly relevant to the anaesthetist, who will appreciate an advanced warning. Patients may be on anticholinesterases (pyridostigmine) or steroids, neither of which should be withdrawn. There is a very high risk of postop ventilatory failure requiring ventilation and/or plasmaphoresis. Less commonly, there may also be a cardiomyopathy. Liaise with the neurologist and with ITU as soon as possible.

Muscular dystrophy

Progressive skeletal deformity causes a restrictive chest problem and coughing is poor due to weakness. Cardiomyopathy is invariably present.

Chapter I.9

PRE-EXISTING PSYCHIATRY

Chapter I.9

PRE-EXISTING PSYCHIATRY

KEY POINTS

Most of the problems posed by patients with psychiatric illness are due
to either their drug regimen or concerns about consent for surgery.
Don't alter psychiatric drug regimens without psychiatric advice.
Study carefully the law concerning consent in mental illness.

Drugs

Benzodiazepines
These are very commonly used, often incorrectly, for insomnia and a variety
of anxiety states. Sudden withdrawal precipitates a nasty syndrome which
looks like a panic attack; severe cases may even fit or become delirious. These
symptoms may develop within a day to a week of withdrawal, depending
upon the half-life of the agent. Prevention is better than cure; continue the
usual medication. If prescribing benzodiazepines you must make it clear to
the patient that they are addictive and are for short-term use only. Do not
include a new prescription for benzodiazepines in the TTOs without
discussing it with the GP.

Antidepressants
The tricyclics and their relations are the mainstay of treatment for
depression. Relevant side-effects include urinary retention, constipation,
blood dyscrasias, electrolyte imbalance, dysrhythmia and confusion. A full
blood count, ECG and electrolytes are needed preoperatively.

A newer class of antidepressant is the SSRIs (selective serotonin re-uptake
inhibitors), which seems to be safer than the tricyclics. However, the same
investigations are indicated.

Monoamine oxidase inhibitors (MAOIs) are often the psychiatrist's last
resort; don't discontinue or change them without consultation. These
patients are forbidden tyramine (and hence alcohol and Marmite – no
wonder they're depressed) and many other drugs. Most importantly they
must not have pethidine or sympathomimetics. Check *all* your prescriptions
against the BNF. (See Chapter I.3.)

Antipsychotics
The typical antipsychotic is the phenothiazine chlorpromazine, which got its
trade name *Largactil* because of its *large* number of *actions*. It acts on
dopaminergic, histamine, serotonin, cholinergic and α-adrenergic pathways.
Small wonder that it has so many side-effects. The ones to watch out for are

Parkinsonism, blood dyscrasias, urinary retention, constipation, hypotension and hypothermia. Its effects are additive with those of other phenothiazines (e.g. prochlorperazine) and other dopamine antagonists (e.g. metoclopramide), so don't write up an anti-emetic just out of habit.

Lithium

Lithium salts are used to stabilize mood in manic and bipolar affective disorders and to treat some forms of depression. The therapeutic window is very narrow (0.4–1.0 mmol/l of Li^+) and toxicity may occur at levels >1.5 mmol/l. The toxicity syndrome shows as mixed cerebellar signs, confusion, coma, convulsions, diarrhoea and vomiting, and may be fatal. Toxicity is precipitated by hyponatraemia, dehydration, pyrexia and loop diuretics. If you have time, it is advisable to measure serum lithium preop (taking the sample within 12 h of last dose). The GP may have a recent result, as it is normal to monitor blood levels. (See Chapter I.3.)

Alcohol

Chronic alcohol abuse leads to many problems (hepatic, neurological, gastrointestinal, haematological, cardiac, pancreatic, malnutrition and diabetes), and each of these must be investigated. As well as dealing with physiological disturbances, you will need to consider the problems of alcohol withdrawal, which is very dangerous indeed. Do not attempt to cure alcoholism in the surgical patient; your job is to prevent withdrawal. The useful drugs to achieve this are: either *alcohol, a benzodiazepine* or *chlormethiazole*. The choice depends on local experience, and advice from a psychiatrist or detoxification specialist is invaluable.

Alcohol can be given by mouth and this might be appropriate for short admissions; only a little is needed (e.g. 1–2 units), you don't have to get them drunk.

Benzodiazepines are the drugs of choice for the emergency treatment of convulsions (diazepam 10–20 mg pr, 10 mg i.v.) and can also be used prophylactically. One regime is to give oral diazepam 30 mg in divided doses on the first day and to reduce by 5 mg/day until a maintenance dose of 10 mg/day is reached.

Chlormethiazole is used by mouth as capsules (192 mg) or as an elixir (50 mg/ml) in a reducing dose, starting with 12 caps (or equivalent) on the first day. Over the first 3 days drop gradually by 50% and over the next week phase out the treatment slowly. Intravenous 0.8% chlormethiazole is titrated against effect (as for alcohol). Run at 5 ml/min until the patient is on the edge of sleep and then reduce to 0.5 ml/min. Reassess frequently, adjusting the flow-rate to achieve a state of calm drowsiness.

Consent

Operations with expressed consent

The vast majority of patients with mental illness remain competent to give their own consent to surgical procedures. This includes most of those who have been admitted under the Mental Health Act (commonly known as being 'sectioned'). **Rule one:** do not erode the autonomy of these, or of any other patients, by failing to explain procedures adequately or by denying the patient an opportunity to make decisions.

Operations under the common law

Some patients, due to acute or chronic confusional states, may be unable to make their own decisions about treatments. The common law imposes upon all doctors a 'duty to care' for such patients. Any treatments, including operations, given in this way must be in the patient's best interest, in accordance with established medical practice and necessary to save life, prevent a deterioration or effect an improvement. If these criteria are met, surgery can be performed without consent. There is no legal basis for the tradition of seeking consent from the next of kin (unless they happen to have the status of legal guardian, e.g. the parents of a minor). However, it is usually appropriate to discuss the proposed treatment with the family and document the interview. **Rule two:** you are allowed to act in the patient's best interest when they are incompetent to give consent; the family do not have the power to either permit or prevent treatment, but it is best to keep them informed and allow them to express their opinions.

Operations for unwilling patients

Any patient who is competent has the absolute right to refuse treatments. Do make sure that the implications of refusal are clear to the patient. Document all discussions clearly and involve your seniors.

Rarely, urgent treatment is refused because of a delusional belief. In this case a conflict of interests arises between your duty to maintain the patient's autonomy and your duty of care towards them. If the patient is clearly incompetent and is putting his safety at immediate risk by refusing treatment, then the duty of care requires you to make the patient safe. This might involve restraint and the use of sedatives. This is scary stuff for the inexperienced; get help from seniors and give thought to an urgent psychiatric consultation. Psychiatrists may be able to help by determining the presence and degree of mental illness, by guiding therapy and by assessing the effect of any illness on competence. **Rule three:** life-saving treatments can be performed against the wishes of an incompetent patient, but never against the wishes of a competent one.

Operations under the Mental Health Act

The act allows only for hospitalization and compulsory treatments for mental illness. **Rule four:** the MHA ('sectioning') does not allow surgery to be performed without consent. Urgent surgery may be allowed under the common law (see above).

Chapter I.10

PRE-EXISTING HAEMATOLOGY

Chapter I.10

PRE-EXISTING HAEMATOLOGY

KEY POINTS

With any complicated blood disease, it is advisable to involve a
  haematologist early.

Anaemias

Anaemias of all aetiologies have in common a reduction in the oxygen-
carrying capacity of the blood. This is compensated by an increase in the
cardiac output, which requires an increase in cardiac work. The main reason
why anaemia matters is that it increases the risk of perioperative ischaemia.

Anaemia is difficult to detect clinically, which is why we screen groups at
risk (see Chapter I.2). Having determined from the full blood count that an
anaemia exists (Hb <12 in males, <10 in females), the next step is to use
indices of erythrocyte size and haemoglobin content to work out the cause.

Hypochromic, microcytic anaemia

This is characterized by small cells, low Hb content (mean corpuscular
volume, MCV <75 fl: mean corpuscular haemoglobin, MCHb <27 pg). This
is most commonly due to chronic blood loss (ulcers, tumours, menorrhagia).
Rarer causes are a failure to absorb oral iron (e.g. post-gastrectomy) or a
failure to utilize iron in Hb production. Simple cases respond to oral iron
therapy (ferrous sulphate 200 mg TDS), which will raise the Hb by 2 g/dl over
a fortnight. Iron can also be given intramuscularly in cases where oral
absorption fails, but this is no quicker in treating anaemia than the oral route.

In a healthy patient with a hypochromic anaemia, surgery can be
performed safely with an Hb as low as 7 g/dl, at the anaesthetist's discretion.
Patients with ischaemic heart disease or other significant illness may need
preoperative transfusion. If transfusion is needed, you can expect one unit of
blood to raise the Hb by 1 g/dl in an average adult (but often by much more
in the elderly). Ideally, transfusion should be completed about 2 days preop
to give time for the stored cells to return to normal oxygen delivery.

Normochromic, normocytic anaemia

This is characterized by normal sized cells, but not enough of them (MCV
76–96 fl: MCHb 27–32 pg). This is most commonly due to the 'anaemia of
chronic disease' and is seen with renal failure, severe connective tissue
diseases like rheumatoid, or carcinoma. In renal failure erythropoetin may be

very effective. These patients rarely need transfusion preoperatively because the anaemia is well compensated for by an increased intracellular 2,3-DPG level which allows the Hb to release its oxygen more easily in the tissues.

Normochromic, normocytic anaemia can also be caused by bone marrow failure in chemotherapy, poisoning, leukaemia or infiltration. Other cell lines are likely to be affected, leading to a pancytopaenia.

Transfusion in renal failure may be harmful, and shouldn't be done without discussion with a renal physician.

Macrocytic anaemia

This condition is characterized by large cells (MCV >96), and is also known as megaloblastic anaemia. These anaemias are the result of either folate or B_{12} deficiencies, which may be due to diet, malabsorption or an increased demand (e.g. pregnancy). Macrocytic anaemias are associated with heart failure; if transfusion is essential use only packed cells and consider using a diuretic. These deficiencies may also cause confusion and spinal cord lesions.

When faced with a new diagnosis of macrocytic anaemia, it is vital to send blood for B_{12} and folate assays and to consult a haematologist. This is because bone marrow biopsy may be indicated before starting treatment and because the incorrect treatment can be harmful. If folate is given before the B_{12} deficiency is corrected it can lead to a worsening of the CNS problems.

B_{12} deficits are treated with hydroxocobalamin. The initial dose is 1 mg i.m.

Bleeding tendencies

Bleeding tendencies acquired during the course of surgery are discussed in Chapter II.7. Patients with bleeding tendencies who present for surgery most commonly have an iatrogenic coagulopathy; pathological coagulopathy is relatively rare. Whatever the nature of the problem, be careful not to make it worse with clumsy use of invasive equipment (e.g. tubes, catheters, drips), by making an excessive number of holes in the patient (i.m. injections) or by incorrect prescription (NSAIDs).

Warfarin

The effects of warfarin therapy are measured by the International Normalized Ratio (INR). An INR of between 2.0 and 4.5 is therapeutic for conditions ranging from DVT prophylaxis to prevention of thrombus formation around mechanical heart valves. Due to difficulty in accurate and rapid control of INR (warfarin is a long-acting drug), it is usual to discontinue warfarin 2–3 days preop and replace it with heparin when major surgery is planned. For minor surgery, it may be acceptable to reduce the dosage of warfarin 2–3 days preop and re-measure the INR to check it is in the lower therapeutic range.

When the INR must be controlled urgently because of trauma or surgery the treatment of choice is FFP. In this situation it is most unlikely that the volume of FFP will pose a problem (the patient is likely to be hypovolaemic). A typical starting dose is 4 units of FFP which has a volume of 800 ml. Always review progress by looking at clinical signs of blood loss and re-measuring the INR. For a catastrophic bleed with raised INR, vitamin K should be considered (5 mg slowly i.v.), but remember that it is slow acting and makes later anticoagulation difficult. There is also a significant incidence of anaphylaxis.

Heparin

Standard, or unfractionated, heparin is the drug of choice for a controllable degree of anticoagulation in the surgical patient. Its very short half-life (~1 h) means that when used i.v. the anticoagulation can be reversed simply by stopping the infusion 3–4 h preop. A typical dose is 1000 units/h i.v. to achieve a 50% prolongation of the partial thromboplastin time (PTT). PTT must be measured at least once a day perioperatively, as individual response is very variable. When restarting warfarin, it is necessary to overlap warfarin and heparin for 2–3 days.

Thrombocytopaenia

A low platelet count (<100 × 10^9/l) is most commonly idiopathic, but may be due to marrow failure or increased consumption. All cases should be discussed with the haematologist. Many of the idiopathic group will respond to steroids. Should a platelet transfusion be essential, each unit of platelets should raise the count by approximately 5 × 10^9/l. The minimum acceptable count for elective invasive procedures is 100 × 10^9/l.

Haemophilia

Haemophiliacs lack factor VIII, and the activity of this factor is measured as a percentage of normal to assess the degree of anticoagulation. The haematologist aims for a factor VIII activity of 100% or better perioperatively. A typical regime is a loading dose of 50 units/kg followed by the same amount per day in divided doses. FFP contains about 1 unit/ml; cryoprecipitate has 25 units/ml. Other drugs that might be used are tranexamic acid or DDAVP.

Christmas disease

Factor IX is replaced using FFP or concentrate and guided by factor IX activity assays.

Von Willebrand's

The principles are as for haemophilia. FFP, DDAVP or cryoprecipitate may be ordered.

Haemoglobinopathy

Haemoglobin structure

Haemoglobin (Hb) contains four protein chains. These are normally of the types α, β, γ or δ and are arranged in pairs. All forms of Hb contain two α chains. HbA is the predominant normal Hb and has two α and two β chains. HbA2 is also normal but present in small amounts; it has two α and two δ chains. HbF is the principal Hb in the fetus, lasting until the age of about 6 months, and has two α and two γ chains.

The types of Hb produced are genetically determined, with contributions from both parents. Thus heterozygotes (e.g. sickle trait) have a mixture of haemoglobins (HbA and HbS), while homozygotes have one predominant type (HbA in normality). In practice, patients unable to make normal HbA partially compensate by increasing the ratio of HbA2 and HbF.

Hundreds of types of abnormal chains are known, but the only important clinical syndromes are sickle cell anaemia and thalassaemia.

Sickle

HbS, sickle haemoglobin, has an abnormality of the β chain which causes the haemoglobin to crystallize under certain conditions (most importantly low oxygen tensions and acidosis). It occurs in Black populations, in the aboriginal peoples of India, in the Middle East and in some Greeks and southern Italians. Heterozygotes form approximately 10% of the black population in the UK; homozygotes about 0.25%.

Detection. Patients with the homozygous state, sickle cell anaemia, will have a well established diagnosis. They are usually extremely knowledgeable about their condition and often the whole family has been tested for sickle trait. Physical signs include: anaemia, splenomegaly in the young, jaundice from haemolysis, growth retardation and evidence of previous infarctions in bone or the CNS.

All surgical patients from the ethnic groups at risk should be tested for sickle trait. This is important so that they can be offered genetic counselling and because some heterozygotes *can* have a sickle crisis (usually when the sickle trait is combined with another abnormal Hb such as HbC). There are no physical signs of the sickle trait. The [Hb] is usually around 11 g/dl, of which about 40% is HbS.

The **Sickledex** test is universally available and is quick to perform. Red cells are exposed to a low pH and a reducing agent, which causes HbS to precipitate. This test shows only the presence or absence of HbS and a positive result must always be followed by an **electrophoresis** to determine which haemoglobins are present and their relative concentrations.

Perioperative management. Those with a sickle trait and *no other haemoglobin-opathy* present no particular problem.

Patients with sickle cell anaemia may present for surgery related to the disease (e.g. with osteomyelitis from bone infarction) or with coincidental pathology. They may be severely anaemic (Hb <6 g/dl). Because sickle is an abnormality of haemoglobin, not of the red cell membrane, the ABO group is not affected and these patients can be cross-matched in the usual way. *All cases must be managed with the advice of a haematologist.*

Preoperatively it may be necessary to transfuse to an Hb of 10 g/dl. Some major surgery may need a partial or complete exchange transfusion.

Operatively, surgeons should be aware that tourniquets can precipitate sickling and that some techniques such as cell-saving autotransfusion are contraindicated.

Postoperatively, your mission is the prevention of a **crisis**. An **infarctive crisis** is due to the formation of clumps of sickled cells obstructing blood vessels. Pain, cold, infection, acidosis and hypoxia are the principal causes. It follows that the patient needs to be well analgesed, kept warm, given oxygen and kept well hydrated. Prophylactic antibiotics and early physiotherapy are routinely used to prevent chest infections. Should a crisis occur, the risk of pulmonary embolus becomes very high and anticoagulation is usually indicated.

Another type of crisis is termed **aplastic**. An increased rate of red cell death or loss following surgery or infection leaves the bone marrow unable to keep up with demand and a life-threatening anaemia develops.

Thalassaemia

This group of haemoglobinopathies occurs in roughly the same ethnic populations as sickle and can occur in the same individual (e.g. HbS–Thal). The classification can be a little confusing, as either the α or β chains may be affected, and sufferers may be either homozygotes or heterozygotes. Heterozygous states result in thalassaemia *minor*. Homozygous states result in thalassaemia *major*. Since α-*thalassaemia major* is incompatible with life, you needn't worry about it. α- or β-*thalassaemia minor* may cause an anaemia but pose no special problem, unless the patient also has the sickle trait.

β-Thalassaemia major (also known as Cooley's anaemia, thalassaemia major) covers a spectrum of severity. At worst, there is severe anaemia and repeated transfusions are needed. Eventually the patient becomes iron overloaded and develops cardiomyopathy and multiple endocrine abnormalities. I would definitely involve the haematologist if I were you.

Polycythaemia

An excess of Hb (>18 g/dl) may be primary, as in polycythaemia rubra vera (PRV), or secondary to an increase in erythropoetin production. The latter is the more common and is usually a response to chronic hypoxia. Rarely a hypernephroma may cause excess erythropoetin secretion.

PRV patients will be known to the haematology department; the most important aspect of their preop preparation is to liaise with the haematologist to arrange venesection preop. Ideally this is done 1–2 days before surgery to avoid adding to perioperative hypovolaemia.

Newly diagnosed polycythaemics should be assumed to have a major respiratory problem until proved otherwise. The history and examination are aimed at detecting heart and chest disease. An ECG, CXR and blood gases are mandatory. Venesection may be indicated preop; discuss this with your friend, the anaesthetist. Postop, these patients are at high risk of DVT and need prophylaxis accordingly.

Chapter I.11

PRE-EXISTING GASTROINTESTINAL AND NUTRITIONAL DISEASE

Chapter I.11

PRE-EXISTING GASTROINTESTINAL AND NUTRITIONAL DISEASE

Obesity

To quantify obesity, the important measurements are weight and height, which are often combined as the *body mass index:*

$$BMI = \text{weight (kg)}/ \text{height}^2 \text{(m}^2\text{)}.$$

Obesity is defined as a BMI of >28, morbid obesity (MO) means a BMI of >35. A BMI of 31 is our upper limit for day-case surgery.

The obese pose special technical problems for the house surgeon and also for the anaesthetist, who will be grateful for an advanced warning.

Cardiovascular system. Hypertension is more common and more difficult to measure, needing an out-sized cuff. Heart failure and ischaemia are also more common, but more difficult to detect. Adipose may mask oedema, and the habitually sedentary may not stress themselves enough to ever suffer angina. The old wives' tale that the obese have 'good engines' because they carry a heavy load around is rubbish. Obesity predisposes to deep vein thrombosis, making early mobilization imperative.

A few of the obese tend to obstruct their airways, particularly at night. This causes hypoxia, raised pulmonary blood pressure, heart failure and polycythaemia. Take a very careful history about snoring, breath-holding at night or day-time drowsiness. If at all suspicious, or if there is polycythaemia, you must send a resting blood gas (breathing air), as this will be very important in deciding on postop oxygen therapy. A raised P_aCO_2 or HCO_3 might indicate the *rare* condition of carbon dioxide retention and be a contra-indication to postop oxygen. Analgesia is also difficult for carbon dioxide retainers as they are easy to over-sedate; get the help of an anaesthetist. A bed on the high-dependency unit is strongly recommended. All the obese need a preop ECG and, if there is any suspicion of carbon dioxide retention or failure, or if major surgery is planned, they will also need a chest X-ray.

Respiratory. The chest is compressed by the mass of tissue around it, making for a small lung volume and a high work of breathing. These patients are prone to chest infections. Preventative measures include nursing the patient upright, sitting out and mobilizing as soon as possible, good analgesia, early physiotherapy and oxygen therapy, especially at night (but see above).

Gastrointestinal. Hiatus hernias, regurgitation and heartburn are common. Continue H_2 blockers or omeprazole perioperatively, but don't give chalky antacids (e.g. magnesium trisilicate) or alginates (e.g. Gaviscon), as the results when these are aspirated are horrific. Prescribe sodium citrate 30 ml PRN instead for symptomatic relief.

Metabolic. Screen for diabetes with urinalysis and blood glucose measurement. Remember the possibility of a temporary insulin dependence.

Practicalities. Avoid intramuscular injections as they are likely to actually be intra-adipose and won't deliver the drug reliably. Intravenous access might be difficult; if you think prolonged i.v. drugs or fluids might be needed, consider a central line at the time of surgery.

Malnutrition

General protein–calorie malnutrition is very common in surgical patients, and may be related to the surgical pathology (malignancies, malabsorptions, pathological fractures) or may be coincidental. Frequently, the malnourished present as emergencies (fractured neck of femur, bowel obstruction) and then their problems are compounded by dehydration, blood loss, electrolyte imbalance or hypothermia. To detect and reverse these problems pre-operatively, the relevant investigations are:

1. *FBC*: to determine anaemia due to iron deficiency, vitamin deficiency or chronic disease. Leukocytopaenia is a sign of malnutrition.
2. *Creatinine/urea/electrolytes*: particularly if there is a history of diarrhoea or vomiting.
3. *Glucose*: you might detect chronic hypoglycaemia due to starvation; paradoxically, when fed adequately these patients may become hyperglycaemic and need insulin.
4. *ECG*: cardiac muscle is weakened along with skeletal muscle; failure and dysrhythmia are more common.
5. *CXR*: preop pneumonia is common due to immunocompromise and weakness. Pulmonary oedema or pleural effusions can be related to hypoalbuminaemia, malignancy or heart failure. Look for secondary malignancies.
6. *LFT/clotting*: hypoalbuminaemia, hypoglobulinaemia and prolonged INR all result from reduced protein synthesis in the malnourished.

Postop, the weakness, immunocompromise and low metabolic rate of these patients makes them prone to infection, poor healing, skin ulceration and hypothermia. Help from physiotherapists, nurses and dieticians is the secret of success. Your role as house surgeon is to be vigilant in detecting infections early, to monitor biochemical changes frequently as feeding is restarted and to avoid iatrogenic problems due to ill-advised use of drugs. These patients generally require lower than usual drug doses (even on a per kg basis); sedation is best avoided and analgesics should be carefully titrated against response. Once again, the intramuscular route is unreliable due to reduced blood flow in muscle.

Upper GI tract problems

Patients may present with a range of problems from indigestion to oesophageal obstruction. Those with severe upper GI tract disease are at risk of malnutrition, chronic bleeding and aspiration pneumonia. The relevant preop investigations are:

1. *FBC*: iron deficiency, malnutrition, rarely Plummer–Vinson syndrome.

2. *LFT, clotting, glucose*: as for malnutrition.
3. *ECG*: symptoms of angina are difficult to distinguish from those of oesophagitis and share the same aetiology (smoking, obesity).
4. *CXR*: any history of choking or chronic cough in patients with oesophageal or laryngeal pathology should lead you to suspect aspiration. Carcinoma of the bronchus can also cause a recurrent laryngeal nerve palsy.

Heartburn and indigestion
Continue or start H_2 antagonists (e.g. ranitidine 150 mg TDS) or omeprazole (20 mg daily). Metoclopramide or cisapride improve stomach sphincter tone and emptying. Particulate antacids and alginates should be stopped and replaced with sodium citrate (see under obesity).

Upper GI bleeding
The principles of care are the same as for bleeding from any other site (see Chapter II.7). Direct control of oesophageal bleeds can sometimes be achieved with a Sengstaken tube. Ranitidine is usually started although it has no action in stopping an existing bleed.

Livers

Don't repeat this at an exam: LFTs are very simple and there are only two diseases of the liver, *acute jaundice* and *liver failure*.

LFTs
Bilirubin is a yellow pigment (normal range <17 micromol/l) whose function is to cause renal failure. *Albumin* is a protein without which you get oedema and ascites. The *INR* is a measure of clotting, which is impaired in liver disease. *Enzymes* (γ-GT, AST, etc.) are not measures of liver function at all, but of liver damage.

Acute jaundice
If a patient turns up for elective surgery and is found to be yellow, you must certainly cancel the case and refer him for diagnosis. More commonly, a patient with jaundice presents for urgent biliary surgery. The main points in this situation are to prevent *renal failure, bleeding* and *hypoxia*.

Renal failure in jaundice is caused by toxins, and the precipitating factor is hypovolaemia. Starting preoperatively and continuing until the jaundice has resolved, you must watch the daily U&Es like a hawk and monitor hourly urine output. Using generous amounts of fluid, you must achieve an output of 1 ml/kg/h. The choice of fluid is not critical in acute obstructive jaundice; these patients have plenty of healthy liver cells and do not cause the fluid balance problems of liver failure (see below). If you are concerned about fluid overload, or if the patient becomes oliguric, start measuring CVP as soon as possible. If the jaundice is severe (>100 micromol/l), mannitol 0.5 g/kg may be given preoperatively as a radical-scavenger and as a diuretic. Don't use diuretics to treat oliguria without CVP measurement; if the patient is hypovolaemic (as is likely), you will put the kidneys at greater risk.

Clotting is deranged in jaundice, as shown by a prolonged INR. Vitamin K is fat soluble and therefore relies on bile salts in the intestine for absorption.

Give phytomenadione 1 mg slowly i.v. preoperatively. This will take 24 h to work, so if there is active bleeding or you need control more quickly give FFP (usually ~5 units) and re-check the INR when finished.

Hypoxia is common postop in jaundiced patients because of increased pulmonary shunt and because of the effects of upper abdominal surgery. Prescribe oxygen for 24 h and for 3 postop nights, and use a pulse oximeter. Good analgesia will also help prevent hypoxia.

Liver failure

Cirrhosis can result from any long-term liver damage but only becomes a problem when the liver fails, leading to *ascites, jaundice* and *encephalopathy*.

- Ascites, effusions and peripheral and pulmonary oedema are a result of salt and water retention, portal hypertension and hypoalbuminaemia.
- Jaundice develops as the liver is unable to cope with a normal excretory load and will worsen with increased haemolysis (e.g. after surgery).
- Encephalopathy, ranging from confusion to coma, is due to neurotoxins such as ammonia which the liver fails to eliminate; the signs are easily confused with those of alcohol withdrawal.

In addition, the circulation is often hyperdynamic, with a tachycardia, vasodilation and hypotension. Cyanosis is common. Portal hypertension leads to oesophageal varices. Diabetes or hypoglycaemia can both be seen. Biochemical abnormalities include hypokalaemia, a low urea and a dilutional hyponatraemia (despite an overall sodium retention).

Clotting is dealt with by replacing clotting factors. Vitamin K is useless. The gastric mucosa should be protected with barrier preparations and H_2 antagonists or omeprazole, although haemorrhage from oesophageal varices is not prevented by these agents.

Renal failure must still be prevented through maintaining a diuresis. Fluid balance in liver failure is discussed in Chapter II.6.

Drugs are unpredictable in their actions due to abnormal protein binding and metabolism. Sedatives must be avoided, and analgesics should be titrated in small doses i.v.

Preventing encephalopathy can be achieved by reducing the amount of protein and nitrogenous breakdown products in the gut. Order a low protein (<20 g/day) diet. Consult a hepatologist who may recommend oral neomycin and lactulose and/or rectal magnesium sulphate.

Lower GI tract problems

Diarrhoea

The principle components lost in diarrhoea are water, sodium, potassium and bicarbonate, resulting in *hypovolaemia, hyponatraemia, hypokalaemia* and *acidosis*. The resuscitation fluid of choice is 0.9% saline with KCl 20–40 mmol/l, depending on serum K^+ results. Acidosis may be treated with bicarbonate (see Chapters II.6 and II.9). Success in resuscitation depends on vigilant monitoring.

Bowel prep

This is an iatrogenic diarrhoea. Hypovolaemia is common. We think it is good practice to put up a drip for 24 h preoperatively and give 2 litres of saline.

Chapter I.12

MISCELLANEOUS PRE-EXISTING CONDITIONS

MISCELLANEOUS PRE-EXISTING CONDITIONS

KEY POINTS

Rheumatoid arthritis is a multi-system disease.
Pregnant patients should not be operated on unless absolutely necessary. Physiological variables are significantly different in late pregnancy. Heavily pregnant women should not lie completely flat.
Anaesthesia and breast feeding need not exclude one another.

Rheumatoid arthritis

This is a common autoimmune disease, primarily affecting the joints, but with a wide variety of extra-articular manifestations. Patients commonly present for orthopaedic procedures, especially joint replacement. Features include:

1. *Articular involvement.* Rheumatoid arthritis may affect any joint, but those of particular interest are the cervical spine and temporomandibular joints. Any patient with restricted or painful neck movements should have a lateral C-spine X-ray. Cervical instability may occur in up to **25%** of rheumatoid patients, and the commonest lesion is atlanto-axial subluxation. Consider applying a semi-rigid collar for the perioperative period.

   Involvement of other joints necessitates careful physical handling, especially when the patient is unconscious. Patients with severe hand disease may not be able to use a conventional patient-controlled analgesia device.

2. *Extra-articular involvement.* Rheumatoid arthritis is a multi-system disease. Be aware that it may affect:

   - *Lungs:* pleural effusions, nodules and pulmonary fibrosis can all occur. Poor exercise tolerance may be masked by the restrictions of joint involvement. A chest X-ray is a justifiable screening test, and respiratory function tests should be done where there is known involvement.
   - *Kidneys:* 25% of patients with rheumatoid arthritis die of renal failure. Kidney disease is the result of both the arthritis, and its treatment (NSAIDs, penicillamine, gold). U&Es should be sent, but may be normal in the presence of significant impairment.
   - *Heart:* involved in 35% of cases, with pericarditis or left ventricular failure. Again, poor exercise tolerance may be masked. Cardiological opinion and/or echocardiography may be indicated in severe cases.

- *Blood*: patients with rheumatoid arthritis are commonly anaemic, either iron deficient or the normochromic 'anaemia of chronic disease'.
- *Nerves*: peripheral neuropathy is common.

Patients with rheumatoid arthritis are at risk of DVT formation.

Pregnancy

OK, it's not a disease. But it's important.

The most common indications for surgery during pregnancy are for abortion, caesarean section and certain obstetric procedures such as insertion of Shirodkar suture. These patients will normally be looked after by people who understand such things.

Occasionally, however, pregnant patients appear on surgical wards for procedures not related to pregnancy. There are a number of special considerations.

- Elective surgery should be avoided if at all possible during pregnancy. Major surgery should be carried out only for maternal survival.
- The risks to the fetus are possible teratogenic effects of anaesthesia-related drugs in the first trimester, and of premature labour in the third. If surgery must be carried out the second trimester is safest.
- Anaesthesia in pregnancy poses special risks to the mother. Failed intubation is more common as a result of physiological changes of pregnancy. After 16 weeks, there is a greater risk of pulmonary aspiration. For this reason, patients are given ranitidine and sodium citrate as a premed.
- Physiological variables alter in pregnancy. Resting respiratory rate and heart rate are higher. Blood pressure is lower (e.g. 90 mmHg systolic may be quite normal). Haemoglobin levels are reduced by up to 20%. Overall blood volume is increased. There is a greatly increased risk of DVT and pulmonary embolus. Raised JVP, systolic murmur (pulmonary flow), third heart sound and peripheral oedema are all normal findings in late pregnancy. Supine hypotension may occur, where the gravid uterus compresses the inferior vena cava when the patient is flat on her back. This can be prevented by nursing the patient on her side or by tilting the mattress to the left with a wedge (available on the labour ward). Hypoxia after surgery is more common. Urine output and maintenance fluid requirements are greater.
- Inform the midwife or obstetrician when a pregnant patient is admitted. This is of particular importance for urgent or major surgery. The presence of a midwife will reassure the patient and provide a source of advice for further monitoring and management.
- Check all prescriptions against the 'prescribing in pregnancy' section of the BNF.

Breast feeding

Nursing mothers who present for surgery are often anxious about the effect of anaesthesia on the baby. Anaesthetic drugs do pass into breast milk, but the levels are too miniscule to pose any threat to the baby. Morphine, diamorphine, paracetamol, ibuprofen, diclofenac, metoclopramide and heparin are also safe.

Drugs which should not be given to lactating mothers

Aspirin:	risk of Reye's syndrome in baby
Atropine:	can cause anticholinergic effects
Barbiturates:	can cause drowsiness in large doses
Chloramphenicol:	can cause bone marrow toxicity in baby
Ciprofloxacin:	large concentrations in breast milk
Tetracycline:	possibility of dental discoloration

Chapter I.13

INFECTION RISK

Chapter I.13

INFECTION RISK

KEY POINTS

Universal precautions are so called because they should be applied for *every* patient.

If you suffer an inoculation injury, you should report it immediately. You do not necessarily need to have an HIV test.

MRSA behaves like any other *Staphylococcus aureus*, except that it is resistant to many antibiotics. Attempts to prevent widespread colonization with MRSA are employed in order to preserve the usefulness of β-lactam antibiotics. Cross-infection can be reduced if you always wash your hands between patients.

Introduction

It is becoming increasingly common for patients with communicable diseases to present for surgery. The most important conditions under this category are HIV, hepatitis B, hepatitis C and the growing problem of MRSA (methicillin-resistant *Staphylococcus aureus*).
There are two priorities:
1. Don't catch any nasty diseases yourself (at least not at work).
2. Don't allow transmission to other patients.

Universal precautions

This is a set of precautions intended to protect staff against blood-borne infections. As the prevalence of agents such as HIV increases, it becomes increasingly pointless to waste time deciding who may be carrying such viruses, and more important to take precautions with *every* patient. The most important measures are:
- Wear gloves whenever contact with bodily fluids is possible.
- Follow sensible practice with sharps. Dispose of them immediately in a sharps bin. Use a tray when putting in a venflon to avoid spiking yourself or someone else. *Never* resheath a needle after taking blood (again, a tray is handy). Always clear up your own sharps.
- Where blood or other fluids are liable to splash about, a mask and eye protection are mandatory.
- Blood-borne viruses do not normally penetrate intact skin, but infection has occurred where contaminated fluid has come into contact with cuts or abrasions, or areas of extensive eczema. Cover all wounds with a waterproof dressing. Those with severe eczema or psoriasis need to take extra care.

HIV

The first case of AIDS was recognized in 1981. Since then the prevalence has increased dramatically. The number of reported cases of AIDS in the UK was 5894 in April 1992. The number of HIV-positive individuals in Britain is not known for sure, but probably exceeds 50 000.

HIV may be present in blood, semen, cerebrospinal fluid and synovial fluid. Saliva, vomit, urine, sputum and sweat are not considered to pose a threat. By 1992 there had been 146 reported cases of occupational transmission of HIV world-wide. A prospective study of transmission following needle stick injury gave the incidence as 0.39%.

Screening of patients for HIV infection does not reduce the incidence of occupational transmission. The existence of the 3-month 'window period' during which an infected individual is yet to produce anti-HIV antibodies, makes a negative result meaningless. HIV tests may not be ordered without the express consent of the patient.

Hepatitis B

Hepatitis B infection is a major global health problem; 2000 cases are reported in Britain each year, though this is probably an underestimate as many cases are asymptomatic. Of those infected, 5–10% go on to be carriers. The carrier state has two forms:

1. Those in whom the hepatitis B surface antigen (HepBsAg) persists for >6 months. These patients are moderately infectious.
2. Those in whom the core antigen (HepBeAg) persists. These individuals have large concentrations of virus in their blood and are highly infectious. They are sometimes called 'super carriers'.

HBV is present in all secretions, though transmission has only firmly been attributed to blood. The risk of transmission following occupational exposure is very much higher than HIV, being in the order of 5–30%.

The most important protection against hepatitis B is vaccination. Proof of immunity against hepatitis B has become a requirement of employment for many health care workers.

Hepatitis C

Previously known as 'transfusion hepatitis', hepatitis C is a blood-borne virus, most commonly associated with blood transfusion. Occupational transmission is rare, but has been reported. Up to 50% of patients infected go on to develop chronic liver disease.

Procedure in the event of inoculation

If you receive a needle stick injury, or are splashed with blood or contaminated fluid, it is essential to report the incident immediately. The best way is to fill in an incident form. Puncture wounds should be squeezed to encourage bleeding, and the wound should be washed thoroughly with soap and water. Splashes into the eyes or mouth should be washed out with clean water.

Subsequent action, such as whether or not blood tests or vaccinations are necessary, should be discussed with the occupational health department at the earliest opportunity. Certain measures, such as use of hepatitis B-specific immunoglobulin or AZT may be required. Don't forget that no-one can make you take an HIV test (or any other test) if you don't want it. Occupational health are there to help you: don't be afraid to use them.

The infected doctor

Transmission of HIV and HBV from doctor to patient has been described. The Health Department has produced detailed advice concerning under what circumstances an infected doctor may continue to practice. Generally speaking, there is no requirement to cease practice, except where 'invasive procedures' are involved. Further advice on what constitutes an invasive procedure should be sought in individual cases, but this normally precludes practising in surgery, obstetrics or dentistry.

MRSA

This is the term for multi-resistant strains of the bacterium *Staph. aureus*, that viewers of the BBC's *Points West* programme will remember as 'The Mystery Killer Virus Code-Named 'Mrs. A'.

MRSA is still just a *Staph. aureus*, and behaves in exactly the same way, except for the fact that it is resistant to all β-lactam antibiotics. There are usually agents to which it is sensitive, but these are more toxic (e.g. vancomycin).

Staph. aureus is found colonizing the respiratory tract of 30–40% of the population. If the rate of colonization of MRSA were allowed to rise unchecked, it would eventually render the penicillins and cephalosporins useless. The acute hospital is at greatest risk of widespread MRSA infections, because of the use of antibiotics, and the opportunities for cross-infection.

The measures taken to control MRSA in any individual hospital are determined according to the local circumstances. Sometimes patients referred from other hospitals that are known to have had outbreaks are routinely isolated until screening swabs are done. For known cases, the normal precautions against cross-infection are used. These include:

1. *Handwashing.* This is the single most important measure, and should be done each time you touch a patient, MRSA or not.
2. *Disposable aprons and gloves.* The greatest value of these more inconvenient measures is to emphasize the need for cleanliness, and reducing the number of casual visitors.
3. *Side wards.* These make isolation measures easier to enforce, and are effective. Some isolation cubicles are designed with unidirectional plenum ventilation.

Chapter II.1

ACUTE PAIN: THE PROBLEM

Chapter II.1

ACUTE PAIN: THE PROBLEM

KEY POINTS

Acute pain is poorly managed.
Pain causes a number of important complications, one of which is death.
Pain scores are useful in measuring the effects of treatment.

Is there a problem?

Yes.

OK, what's the problem?

I'll tell you. An important report commissioned jointly by the Royal College of Surgeons and the College of Anaesthetists in 1990, concluded that: "...the current management of acute pain in the perioperative period stinks."

Well, they didn't exactly use those words, but that was the gist of it. Since then many surveys and audit projects have confirmed that postoperative pain is very commonly left untreated, and that those to whom the responsibility falls to manage this pain are undertrained and ill-informed.

There are a number of important reasons for this state of affairs:

1. *Ignorance.* Things are probably changing for the better, but acute pain control has not typically been a priority for medical school curricula.
2. *Fear.* Everyone is taught about all the hideous side-effects of analgesics, no-one is taught the equally hideous side-effects of pain.
3. *Patients.* Patients don't exactly do themselves any favours here, either. Many members of the stoical older generation expect to be in pain, fear the side-effects of analgesics just like their doctors, and tend to suffer in silence. This is why it has taken us so long to realise that there is a problem.
4. *Attitude.* Ignorance of acute pain management encourages the attitude that the patient who says he's still in pain despite a generous 25 mg of pethidine, must be faking or a junkie or something.
5. *Masking of symptoms.* This is a common excuse for leaving a patient in screaming agony. Apart from the initial assessment of the acute admission (possibly), there is no evidence that any technique of pain control results in delayed or missed diagnoses, provided any worsening of pain is met with appropriate assessment before analgesic medication is altered. 'Breakthrough pain' in a previously comfortable patient is an important warning sign.

These chapters give a basic grounding in acute pain management. It is assumed that the cause of the pain is known, as is usual postoperatively. This is not a discussion of the use of the symptom of pain as a diagnostic tool, and indeed that information belongs in a textbook of surgery.

What is paramount is that you **identify causes of pain that need a different form of intervention (i.e. an operation).** You will not be thanked for providing perfect analgesia for a patient's ischaemic leg pain if you do not also recognize that the definitive management is surgery.

Consequences of pain

It ought to be enough that pain is unpleasant, for us to want to treat it properly. There are, however, many important complications of acute pain:
1. *Psychological*: it hurts.
2. *Secondary psychological*: untreated pain leads to anxiety, fear, depression and even overt paranoia.
3. *Respiratory*: hugely important. People who cannot cough, take a deep breath, or tolerate chest physiotherapy because of pain will retain secretions, get pneumonia, become hypoxic and die. This is most relevant for pain near the diaphragm (i.e. abdominal and thoracic wounds). Pain anywhere causes tachypnoea, increases work of breathing and may worsen bronchospasm.
4. *Cardiovascular*: the haemodynamic responses to pain are tachycardia and hypertension, which increase myocardial oxygen consumption, and decrease myocardial oxygen delivery. These same responses are implicated in the development of myocardial ischaemia, infarction and cerebrovascular events.
5. *Other*: pain limits mobilization. This leads to longer hospital stay and all the complications of immobility such as deep vein thrombosis and pressure sores. Pain increases intracranial pressure, which is bad for the injured brain.

Pain measurement

Until someone invents the Pain-O-Meter™, we are reliant on our patients to warn us of the presence and severity of pain. Attempts to find objective measures of pain, particularly in physiological responses like tachycardia, are extremely unreliable, so **pain is what the patient tells you it is**.

The simplest pain measure is the visual analogue scale (VAS) or pain score. The agonized patient is asked for a number or a word (from a limited choice) which best describes the pain. The scale may be 'none–mild–moderate–severe–Aaaaarrrgh!', but I have always found the score from 0 (no pain) to 10 (the worst pain imaginable) to be most useful.

I would encourage you to ask patients for pain scores whenever you are asked to deal with a pain problem, both before and after any intervention, and document it.

You should understand that a single pain score is meaningless, in that it is influenced by many emotional and cognitive factors, but a *series* of pain scores is extremely useful in assessing response to treatment. Reducing a pain score from 7 to 3 is a job well done. Pain scores cannot be used to compare one patient with another, nor will they tell you how much morphine to give. As with many things, careful titration of therapy against response, with frequent reassessment, is the key.

Chapter II.2

Pain Management: the Drugs

Chapter II.2

PAIN MANAGEMENT: THE DRUGS

KEY POINTS

The important properties of all opioids are the same. They all cause analgesia, nausea and vomiting, and respiratory depression.

Opioids are **safe**. There is a wide therapeutic window, and a specific antagonist. They have been in use for thousands of years. **Pain** is dangerous.

None of the commonly used opioids is any 'stronger' than the others.

Patients given opioids appropriately for acute pain do **not** become addicted.

Non-steroidal anti-inflammatory drugs are extremely useful adjuncts to postoperative pain management. They have important side-effects however: bronchospasm, gastrointestinal bleeding, renal damage, platelet inhibition and drug interactions.

Opioids: general points

The opioids are the mainstay of management of acute pain. (An opi*ate* is a derivative of opium, an opi*oid* is anything that acts at opioid receptors, and includes synthetic drugs like pethidine. They are also called narcotic analgesics.)

These drugs have a number of things in common, sometimes called the cardinal properties of opioids. They all cause analgesia, nausea and vomiting, respiratory depression and addiction.

1. *Analgesia.* Obviously the reason we use them. It is a common misunderstanding to consider one drug to be 'stronger' than another. The maximum analgesic effect of morphine is the same as that of pethidine, omnopon or diamorphine. Diamorphine is more *potent*, but that simply means you need fewer milligrams to achieve the same effect. Dose requirements vary enormously, and cannot be easily predicted by weight.

2. *Nausea and vomiting.* This is common, and this is the reason why you should write up an anti-emetic with your opioid (see Chapter II.5).

3. *Respiratory depression.* The most important and potentially dangerous side-effect. It is common to all opioids and, regardless of the claims of some manufacturers, it always occurs in proportion to the analgesic effects. There are a number of important points:

   • Under normal circumstances, patients do not stop breathing without first becoming comfortable. This is the 'therapeutic window' and for opioids, it is fairly wide.

- The simplest way to assess respiratory depression is by counting respiratory rate, less than eight breaths per minute being a worrying sign. However, this is unreliable, as patients often breathe adequately at lower rates (especially when asleep).
- Never use a pulse oximeter to detect respiratory depression. Hypoxia is an extremely late sign, especially if the patient is breathing oxygen.
- Respiratory depression is accompanied by somnolence. In its early stages, patients 'forget' to breathe, and can be reminded with a little prod. Patients who are wide awake are unlikely to have opioid-related respiratory depression, whatever their respiratory rate.
- Respiratory depression caused by opioids is managed with small, incremental doses of naloxone, for example 0.2 mg i.v. Naloxone has a short duration of action (~10 min), so repeated doses may be required.

4. *Addiction*. No-one would deny that opioids have the capacity to cause addiction. Fear of this side-effect, however, is the single stupidest reason not to treat pain adequately. If you learn nothing else from this book, understand that **patients given opioids appropriately when in acute pain do NOT become addicted**. Reassure your patients of this fact, too. Patients who need massive doses of opioid can easily be weaned from it as the source of the pain recedes.

People who take opioids for *fun* get addicted.

It is important to realize that the dose requirements vary enormously, and depend on many factors such as severity of pain, age, prior opioid use, psychological factors and weight. Doses may have to be adjusted dramatically for some patients.

Apart from these common properties, there are a number of differences between the available opioids, such as speed of onset, duration of action, smooth muscle effects, elimination, and histamine release. The choice of opioid is determined by the side-effect profile and pharmacokinetic factors.

There are a million and one opioids available, but it is better to become familiar with a small number of favourites. I am going to recommend just three: morphine, diamorphine and pethidine.

Morphine

Morphine is an excellent drug, and dirt cheap. It has a fast onset when given i.v. and a duration of action of about 4–6 h. It can be given orally (as an elixir or slow release preparation such as MST), i.m. or i.v. It has a useful cough-suppressant effect.

Side-effects include delayed gastric emptying and constipation. It may cause spasm of the sphincter of Oddi. It causes histamine release, which may cause bronchospasm in asthmatics. It is converted to an active metabolite, morphine-6-glucuronide which is excreted in the urine. This may accumulate in renal failure. The dose is whatever that patient needs to become comfortable. In practice, a typical i.m. prescription might be 10 mg 3-hourly PRN.

Diamorphine

Diamorphine (heroin) is diacetyl morphine, and is basically a pro-drug for morphine and hence shares most of its properties. It is much more fat soluble than morphine, so has a more rapid onset. An i.m. dose might be 5–10 mg 3-hourly PRN.

Pethidine

Pethidine is included in this list mainly because it lacks histamine-related side-effects, and is safe in asthma. It causes less constipation than morphine, but does not suppress the cough reflex. It has significant anticholinergic properties (and does not constrict the pupils like other opioids). It may cause less spasm at the sphincter of Oddi.

Its main disadvantage is its shorter duration of action than morphine (~2 h). It has a reputation for a higher incidence of nausea and vomiting. Its principal metabolite, norpethidine, can cause serious excitatory neurological effects and can accumulate when large doses (typically >1000 mg/day) are used. A typical dose regimen for an adult might be 75–100 mg i.m., 2-hourly PRN.

Others

The choice of opioids is wider than you need. The following are also commonly used:

- *Papaveretum* (Omnopon) is a mixture of all the water-soluble constituents of opium. It contains morphine, papaverine and codeine. It basically behaves like morphine, although it may be more sedating. It used to contain noscapine, a substance implicated in birth defects. Unfortunately, 'new' noscapine-free omnopon is more expensive. It is presented in ampoules containing 15.4 mg, which can be a pain for the nurses (and thus to you as well) if it isn't written up correctly.

  This curious figure is chosen because it is equivalent to 10 mg of morphine, and this is the point: papaveretum is a perfectly good drug, but it is just a complicated way of giving morphine.

- *Fentanyl* is a clean, short-acting drug used mainly in anaesthesia, but may appear on the wards in an epidural solution (see Chapter II.4).

- *Codeine* is less effective than other drugs because of weak receptor binding. It is sometimes used in situations where opioid side-effects would be undesirable. (e.g. head injuries), but this is not terribly logical. (see Chapter II.4). It doesn't cause side-effects because it doesn't *work*, at least not for severe pain. Codeine is found in many oral preparations which are useful in mild to moderate pain. Dihydrocodeine ('DF118') is claimed to be more effective than codeine, but the evidence is thin.

- *Buprenorphine* is an unusual drug. It is a partial agonist, which means, among other things, that there is a 'ceiling' to its analgesic effect. In addition, it binds unusually strongly to opioid receptors. This means that if you give a dose and it is not effective, it is difficult to displace it with a more effective drug like morphine. Also, if a patient suffered respiratory depression as a result of buprenorphine, it would be extremely hard to reverse with naloxone. It is given by the sublingual route which, being more reliable than intramuscular absorption in shocked young soldiers, is the reason it has found favour with the British Army for battlefield use. This route of administration confers little benefit in the hospital setting, however. It causes a great deal of nausea and vomiting, and, generally speaking, this is a drug to avoid.

Non-steroidal anti-inflammatory drugs

These drugs have a number of properties including analgesic, antipyretic and anti-inflammatory actions. They are very valuable as analgesics in properly selected postoperative patients. Since their mode of action (peripheral inhibition of prostaglandin synthesis) is completely separate from that of the opioids (central receptor agonists), they are safe to use in combination with opioids. As supplementary analgesics, they reduce the requirement for opioids and thus reduce the risk of opioid-induced side-effects. The indications for these drugs are:

- sole therapy for mild to moderate pain;
- in combination with other techniques for moderate to severe pain;
- reduction of fever;
- reduction of inflammation.

The non-steroidals have a list of important side-effects. They are so effective in postoperative pain relief, however, that they should be used in **every** case where contraindications do not exist.

The top five problems with non-steroidal anti-inflammatory drugs are:

1. *Gastric irritation*: occurs with all the NSAIDs in differing degrees. It is due to inhibition of prostaglandins regulating the secretion of gastric acid and therefore is a hazard *whatever the route of administration*. NSAIDs are contraindicated for patients with a history of gastric or duodenal ulcers, or with any other predisposition to upper GI tract bleeding. To minimize this problem, always prescribe NSAIDs to be taken with food. Misoprostol is a prostaglandin preparation which can be taken orally with NSAIDs and reduces the risk of gastric ulceration.

2. *Renal effects*: include a reduction in blood flow, a retention of sodium and water, and chronic renal damage in chronic users (i.e. arthritis sufferers). Use these drugs with caution in anyone with renal disease, hypovolaemia, hypertension or gout, and check U&Es frequently.

3. *Platelet inhibition*: This only becomes a problem postoperatively in people with reduced platelet counts, platelets that are already dysfunctional (e.g. in uraemia or after cardiopulmonary bypass) or who have large raw areas to bleed from. You will not earn many points for inhibiting platelet function after a partial hepatectomy, splenorrhaphy or intracranial surgery, for instance.

   Please remember that platelet function is not necessarily reflected by the platelet count; you should discontinue NSAIDs in anyone who shows clinical evidence of a bleeding problem, regardless of laboratory results (Chapter II.7). Bleeding considered to be due to platelet dysfunction should be treated with platelet transfusion.

4. *Bronchospasm*: smooth muscle tone in the airways is also influenced by prostaglandins. A very alarming syndrome of life-threatening bronchospasm associated with aspirin intolerance and nasal polyps has been reported recently. It is certainly safest to avoid all NSAIDs in asthmatics or those with nasal polyps, unless they have used them before without a problem. These drugs are strongly contraindicated in the presence of active bronchospasm.

5. *Drug interactions*: by far the most important of these is an increase in the anticoagulation during warfarin therapy. This is another strong contra-indication.

There is a large number of these drugs available, most of which are indistinguishable in terms of side-effects or efficacy (despite the manufacturers' claims). The following are listed as examples because they are in common use or have particular advantages in routes of administration.

Many NSAIDs (e.g. indomethacin) are primarily anti-inflammatory and have little to offer as postoperative analgesics.

Aspirin
Antipyretic, anti-inflammatory and analgesic in doses of 500–1000 mg 4- to 6-hourly orally, aspirin is now little used as a postoperative analgesic because other agents give better analgesia with fewer side-effects. Many patients are admitted taking low-dose aspirin for other indications, which makes the use of other NSAIDs undesirable. Aspirin is now absolutely contraindicated for children because of the risk of Reye's syndrome. Paracetamol or ibuprofen are suitable alternatives as analgesics and antipyretics.

Ibuprofen
Ibuprofen is a typical NSAID for oral use. At equianalgesic doses with aspirin it causes fewer side-effects. The dose is 200–400 mg 4- to 8-hourly. The commonest problems are gastric irritation, dizziness, rashes and tinnitus.

Diclofenac (Voltarol)
Diclofenac is commonly used as a perioperative analgesic. It is available as oral (including slow-release), injectable and rectal preparations. The maximum daily dose is 150 mg by any of these routes. The i.m. injections are notoriously painful and have no advantage over the suppository. Voltarol suppositories are now available for children, at a dose of 1–3 mg/kg/day.

Ketorolac
Ketorolac is in vogue with anaesthetists because it is a powerful analgesic (equivalent to 10 mg of morphine) and is available as an injectable. As an i.m. injection it is not unduly painful and it can also be given i.v.. The dosage is under review, but at the time of writing is 10 mg i.v. followed by 30 mg, or 30 mg i.m., at 4- to 6-hourly intervals. The total daily dose should not exceed 90 mg.

Paracetamol and combination pills

The very low risk of side-effects and high efficacy of paracetamol as an analgesic and antipyretic make it the commonest analgesic in use. It is given orally in doses of 500–1000 mg 4- to 6-hourly. Elixirs are available which are very useful for children (15 mg/kg 4- to 6-hourly). Suppositories come in a range of strengths and are given in the same dosage. A particular advantage of paracetamol is that it can be given in conjunction with NSAIDs. Paracetamol does not share the problems of the NSAIDs listed above, and allergies to it are rare. High doses are hepatotoxic and it should be avoided in severe liver disease.

There are a variety of combination preparations that contain paracetamol. The commonest are:
- Co-proxamol: contains dextropropoxyphene 32.5 mg with paracetamol 325 mg.
- Co-dydramol: contains dihydrocodeine 10 mg with paracetamol 500 mg.
- Co-codamol: contains codeine 8 mg with paracetamol 500 mg.

These drugs are useful for mild to moderate pain, and there is little to choose between them. They are a safe alternative when non-steroidals are contraindicated. Note that all these preparations contain opioids, and opioid side-effects are a possibility, particularly in overdose. They all cause constipation. The dosage is determined principally by the paracetamol component of the compound preparation, which should not exceed 50 mg/kg/day. A typical prescription for any of them is two tablets 6-hourly.

Secondary analgesics

Not all drugs that relieve pain are in themselves true analgesics; some act by a secondary effect in modifying the painful pathological process. For instance anti-muscarinic drugs such as hyoscine may reduce pain from gastrointestinal tract spasm, and benzodiazepines have a weak muscle relaxant action which may improve pain associated with skeletal muscle contraction. The anxiolytic effects of benzodiazepines may be useful, but only if anxiety is a major component of the pain state, and this is not usually the case. All too often, benzodiazepines are used inappropriately, the result being an unduly sedated patient who remains in pain. **As a rule, treat pain with analgesics, not sedatives**.

Chapter II.3

SIMPLE ANALGESIC TECHNIQUES

Chapter II.3

Simple Analgesic Techniques

Key Points

PRN medication is inappropriate for severe or long-lasting pain.

Try to include a regular element to any postoperative pain prescription.

Give non-steroidal anti-inflammatory drugs to everyone for whom they are not contraindicated. The combination of NSAIDs and opioids is particularly effective.

Intramuscular medication has many disadvantages, but may be used if you anticipate that only one or two doses will be necessary.

Patients are easier to keep comfortable if you take the time to titrate a controlled i.v. loading dose first.

Intravenous infusions can be effective, but require a loading dose, and close monitoring. Patient-controlled analgesia is generally preferred.

Non-drug analgesia

Don't forget that effective analgesia can sometimes be achieved without the use of drugs. Perhaps the best example is the use of traction or splinting in limb injuries. A properly fitted plaster of Paris can work wonders following fracture or for joint effusion.

Much has been written on the power of placebo to treat pain. Placebo can be used in controlled trials following full informed consent from the patient, but to give a placebo to a patient who believes he is receiving an analgesic is deceitful, and could expose you to the risk of litigation. There are many ways to deal with the troublesome drug-seeking patient (see Chapter II.4), but this is not one of them.

The analgesic ladder

This is an important but extremely limited concept, which is traditionally taught as the be-all and end-all of acute pain management.

The analgesic ladder approach identifies the commonly available drugs in order of 'strength' (e.g. paracetamol, aspirin, voltarol, co-proxamol, dihydrocodeine, morphine, diamorphine). You start at the bottom and work up until pain is alleviated.

Viewed at its simplest, this is entirely valid: you wouldn't wade in with i.v. diamorphine at the first sign of a mild headache. There are however serious flaws.

- This approach places all the emphasis on the choice of drug, and not the method of delivery. Much evidence from recent years, particularly from studies into patient-controlled analgesia, points to exactly the reverse being important.
- The ladder does not hold for all situations, for example NSAIDS may be more effective than opioids for bony pain (e.g. in fractures or bone metastases).
- It ignores the advantages of combination therapy (see below).
- It simply doesn't apply to the postoperative patient.

Enteral therapy

This is the simplest form of pain management. It includes oral, rectal or nasogastric administration. This is the preferred method of drug delivery wherever possible, being both safe and convenient. Even severe pain, if it is stable and long-lasting, can be managed via the oral route.

Oral therapy requires a functioning gut, and is thus not always available postoperatively. Rectal medication can still be given, but bear in mind that the pain caused by manoeuvring into the suppository position may outweigh the benefits (e.g. in a patient with multiple injuries).

Often, the bioavailability of oral drugs is less than the parenteral preparation, and people tend to get disproportionately excited about this. If the oral bioavailability of a drug is 1/3, it just means you give three times as much for the same effect. It should *not* affect your choice of agent. When converting parenteral therapy to oral, check the dose adjustment (see 'Action plan for analgesic drugs', p. 259).

Medication down the nasogastric tube requires a liquid preparation. There are a number available: paracetamol elixir (250 mg / 5 ml), aspirin (dispersible), co-codamol (dispersible), ibuprofen (Brufen syrup or dispersible granules), naproxen (Naprosyn syrup), dihydrocodeine elixir (10 mg/5 ml), morphine elixir (e.g. Oramorph, various strengths), MST (as dispersible granules).

Intramuscular therapy

The i.m. route has seen long service on surgical wards, and is most commonly used for opioids. It is simple, adaptable and often effective. Its disadvantages are however, numerous.
- First, it is usually prescribed on a PRN basis, which is bad (see below).
- Intramuscular therapy is time-consuming and labour-intensive because of the controls on the use and storage of narcotic analgesics
- Intramuscular injections hurt; the fear of needles often prevents patients from asking for analgesia.
- Once the injection is given, there is a delay, after which relatively high plasma levels of drug are achieved. During this phase, side-effects (nausea, respiratory depression) are likely. This period is followed by a fall in plasma levels during which the pain returns until another injection is requested. The patient thus bounces between too high and too low a plasma level and so experiences alternating side-effects and pain (see Figure II.3.1).
- Absorption of drugs from the muscle is variable at best. In shocked or

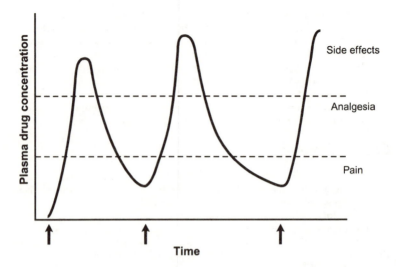

Figure II.3.1.   A graph of plasma drug concentration vs. time during repeated intramuscular injections.

hypovolaemic patients the perfusion of muscle is reduced, resulting in delayed absorption until the shock state is corrected when too much drug may be released. A similar problem is seen when drug is stored in the inactive muscle of immobile patients, only to be released when the muscle is used again on mobilizing.

Some of these problems can be overcome by regular (as opposed to PRN) injections, but if such prolonged analgesia is anticipated you should consider another route. The i.m. route is contraindicated in severe coagulation disturbance and in the shocked patient.

Intramuscular injections of opioids remain useful and appropriate in those patients who have moderate pain and who are expected to rapidly progress to oral medication. If your patient needs more than one or two i.m. doses, think of another regimen.

The combination approach

The addition of an NSAID to an opioid regimen leads to a significant reduction in the required dose of opioid and the incidence of side-effects.

The benefits of this combination are such that you should ensure that **every** patient in whom the drugs are not contraindicated receives a regular non-steroidal, whatever else they are being given for pain. (The contra-indications, in case you'd forgotten, are: asthma, ulcers, renal impairment, platelet dysfunction, warfarin therapy.)

PRN vs. regular medication

PRN stands for 'pro re nata', which is Latin for 'absolutely useless pain management'.

OK, I made that up, but you get the point. If you *know* your patient is going to suffer pain, it is illogical to write all the pain medication up 'as required'. For a start, it requires pain to return before therapy is given. The patient has to *ask* for analgesia from overstretched nurses who are hurtling past him so fast they are red from the Doppler effect. There is good evidence that only a fraction of the medication prescribed as PRN is actually given.

With the exception of very mild short-lived pain, try to have a **regular** element to any pain prescription you write, with a PRN **rescue** medication. For example, for a hernia repair:

> Voltarol 50 mg orally tds,
>
> plus   morphine 10 mg i.m., 3-hourly PRN.

You should write a stop or review date, to ensure that these drugs don't continue longer than necessary. In my experience, however, patients will decline the medication if it is not required. The important thing is that they were *offered* it.

Intravenous infusions

Intravenous infusions were used more widely before the advent of patient-controlled analgesia, but are still in use. They have a number of advantages over intermittent i.m. administration. The aim is that once the patient is properly loaded, analgesic drug is trickled in at the same rate as it is being eliminated, thus producing steady-state effective analgesia.

The problem is that it is very difficult to judge the correct infusion rate. Too slow, and the patient will become uncomfortable again. Too fast, and the patient will become steadily more narcotized, often without being noticed until it is too late.

It is therefore safer to set the infusion rate too low to start with. When the patient becomes uncomfortable again, it is essential to give a small bolus first, then increase the infusion rate. One of the most dangerous regimens of all is the infusion started *without* a loading dose. In this situation, the doctor is repeatedly called back to see the patient, and at each visit (unless he decides the patient is faking) he increases the infusion rate. With this process, it takes about 6 h for the patient to become comfortable (i.e. loaded), and about 45 min more for them to become dead (see Figure II.3.2).

Loading doses

You will hear that even the most advanced and complex pain regimens are hopeless without an initial loading dose. Giving a loading dose is an important technique to learn. It takes 10–15 min, but if done properly it will save you and your patient countless hours of aggro later.

Loading doses are given *intravenously*. Ask the patient for a pain score. Then give a small dose of your chosen opioid (e.g. 2 mg morphine or 10 mg pethidine). Wait a few minutes, and ask again. This is another example of a servo loop (see Figure II.3.3), that is assessment–therapy–reassessment. Continue this process (allowing time for the dose to act at each cycle) until you have made a significant difference to the pain score, or (unusual) the patient begins to get somnolent. It is probably a good idea to have an ampoule of naloxone (0.4 mg) handy, but if you do it properly it won't be required.

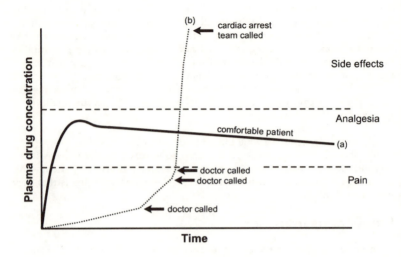

Figure II.3.2   A graph of plasma drug concentration vs. time during intravenous infusion. (a) With initial loading dose. (b) Without initial loading dose.

Other simple techniques

The subcutaneous route is extremely useful, combining some of the advantages of i.v. administration, with a degree of safety and convenience. This is preferred in terminal care (see the Final Chapter).

Inhalational analgesia is used for short-lived severe pain, for example for painful dressing changes or uterine contractions. Entonox® is a 50:50 mixture of oxygen and nitrous oxide, which is supplied with a demand valve breathing system for this purpose.

Choice of technique

With the variety of techniques of pain control at your disposal, it ought to be possible to keep the vast majority of your patients comfy. One remaining difficulty, however, is to predict the duration and severity of postoperative pain, and to choose an appropriate technique. Who would guess, for example, that total knee replacement would be so much more painful than total hip replacement, as is the case?

The only answer to this is experience, unfortunately, so do not be afraid to be flexible, or to seek advice when in doubt.

The table below gives a framework to plan for your patients analgesic needs.

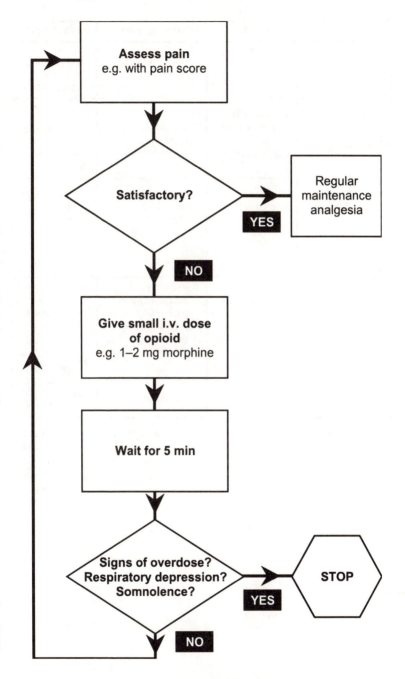

Figure II.3.3.   Loading dose flow chart.

	Mild pain	**Moderate pain**	**Severe pain**
Very short term (<1 h)		i.v. bolus i.m. bolus N_2O	General or regional anaesthetics
Short term (1–12 h)	Simple oral preparations (e.g. paracetamol)	i.m. bolus i.v. bolus Single-shot nerve blocks	i.v. titrated boluses Regional or peripheral blocks
Medium term (1 day–1 week)	Oral preparations	i.m. intermittent (limited to 1 day only) i.v. infusions PCA Epidural	i.v. infusions PCA Regional blocks
Prolonged (>1 week)	Oral preparations	Convert to long-term oral agents after initial infusion, PCA or epidural	High dose oral long-term agents (e.g. MST) Subcutaneous infusions Transdermal opioids Pain clinic procedures

Notes: consider adding NSAIDS in any situation; consider seeking expert help (i.e. anaesthetics, acute pain service, pain clinic) for shaded areas.

Chapter II.4

ADVANCED ANALGESIC TECHNIQUES

Chapter II.4

ADVANCED ANALGESIC TECHNIQUES

KEY POINTS

Patient-controlled analgesia is safe, effective, versatile, popular, cost-effective and non-labour intensive, but not foolproof.

Epidural analgesia probably provides the best analgesia available, but poses special risks.

Pain management in shock, respiratory disease, head injury, drug addicts and children is difficult, but avoiding the issue is not the answer. Acute pain teams can help.

Keep an eye out for the patient who is suffering from neurogenic pain, which is different in character from the usual pain. Neurogenic pain does not respond to opioids.

Patient-controlled analgesia

The first commercially available patient-controlled analgesia device (the Cardiff palliator) was developed in 1976. However, this technique has only recently been available on a wide scale.

There are two fundamental problems with acute pain management in the postoperative period.

1. There is an enormous variation in the analgesic requirements following similar operations, for both pharmacokinetic and psychological reasons.
2. The patient is the only person who knows how much pain the patient is suffering.

The technique of patient-controlled analgesia is the only way to address both these problems. It is unparalleled in its:

- **Safety**. When set up properly, overdose is extremely unlikely, barring a fault in the pump. As the levels increase, the patient becomes increasingly disinclined to trigger further doses. Opioid-related side-effects are fewer, because analgesia is more closely matched to the pain.
- **Efficacy**. Patient-controlled analgesia has been shown to be highly effective for almost all kinds of acute pain. Giving the patients control over their own medication has a powerful psychological effect, which in itself reduces the analgesic requirement.

If patient-controlled analgesia is started after an appropriate loading dose, the patient will be able to maintain a drug level within the therapeutic window, avoiding both pain and side-effects (see Figure II.4.1).

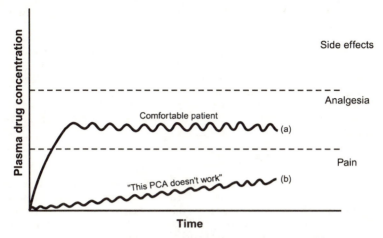

Figure II.4.1. A graph of plasma drug concentration vs. time during patient-controlled analgesia. (a) With initial loading dose. (b) Without initial loading dose.

A patient-controlled analgesia pump consists of a programmable syringe driver with a hand-held trigger switch. It is used to control the i.v. delivery of the chosen analgesic (usually morphine, diamorphine or pethidine). When the device is set up the following parameters are chosen:

1. *Drug concentration*: typically morphine 1 mg/ml; pethidine 10 mg/ml.
2. *Bolus dose*: the amount of drug received with each push of the button. Typical values are 1–2 mg morphine or 10 mg pethidine.
3. *Lockout interval*: this is the key safety feature of patient-controlled analgesia. Once a dose is given, there follows a period of time during which requests for further doses are denied, called the 'lockout interval'. This prevents the patient from taking a second dose before the effect of the first is felt. The time chosen varies according to the size of the bolus and the nature of the drugs, but is usually 5–10 min.
4. *Continuous infusion*: this enables an infusion to be given on top of the bolus doses. This was intended to provide basal analgesia whilst the patient sleeps. Studies on elective surgery have shown that background infusions do not improve the quality of analgesia, but increase the incidence of side-effects. This setting is usually zero, therefore.
5. *Maximum dose*: can be set, but usually isn't.

Although patient-controlled analgesia has a good safety record, it is not foolproof. Fatal accidents continue to occur, for example:

- Programming errors: if you set the pump to deliver 100 mg of morphine at each press of the button, an accident will happen. In most hospitals, the pumps may only be tampered with by certain personnel (usually anaesthetists), except in order to change the syringe. As with any drug, meticulous checking of the programme against the prescription and the solution are important safeguards.
- Other people hitting the button. The safety of patient-controlled analgesia relies on the button being pressed by the patient. NCA (nurse-controlled analgesia), DCA (doctor-controlled analgesia) and

MJFNTSCA (Mrs-Johnson-from-number-twenty-seven-controlled analgesia), are not safe alternatives.
- Pump malfunctions. Rare but not impossible.

Patient-controlled analgesia is suitable for acute pain of any cause or duration, provided the patient is capable of operating the handset and understanding the idea, and provided that staff have received adequate training in looking after the pump.

A number of special triggering devices are available for those physically unable to press the normal handset, for example because of arthritis or amputation.

Epidural analgesia

Epidurals have been in use in postoperative pain management for 20 years. In spite of this, they are the source of continuing controversy, and wide variations in practice exist. Enthusiasts (like us) believe that a correctly sited epidural provides the most effective pain relief available, contributes to lower morbidity and leads to fewer side-effects than other techniques. In some hospitals, however, they are banned on the general wards and confined to ITU.

You may be asked to refill epidural syringes, and you may be the first person asked to deal with epidural problems (the second line being some bad-tempered anaesthetic SHO). I hope the following will demystify the subject somewhat.

Pharmacology
The following drugs are used:
- Local anaesthetic. When local is injected, it blocks nerve roots causing sensory and motor block in the areas supplied by those roots. This is what we do when operations are done under epidural.
- Opioids, which act on opioid receptors in the spinal cord. There is much debate about which drug is best. No need to bore you with that here.
- A combination of the two. This is the commonest choice for post-operative analgesia. Normally opioid (fentanyl, morphine or diamorphine) is added to a weak solution of local anaesthetic (e.g. 0.125% bupivacaine). The analgesia is provided mainly by the opioid, and normally the solution does not of itself cause motor or sensory block, or hypotension.

Uses
Epidurals are most useful for:
- thoracotomy or major laparotomy incisions, major vascular surgery;
- major lower limb surgery;
- multiple rib fractures or flail chest;
- high risk patients, especially with respiratory or ischaemic heart disease;
- cancer pain and terminal care.

Adverse effects
The list of problems is long, but serious incidents are rare.
1. *Respiratory depression.* This may occur as a result of opioid spreading up via the CSF to the respiratory centre. It may be that this particular risk

has been overestimated. The diagnosis and management is the same as for respiratory depression from opioids given by other routes.

2. *Hypotension.* This can certainly occur, as a result of vasodilation, which leads to an effective hypovolaemia.

    Management of epidural-related hypotension is, in the first instance, a fluid bolus. There is usually no need to stop the infusion. Do *not* assume that hypotension is always due to the epidural alone, because in practice there is nearly always another cause (e.g. bleeding or fluid losses).

    Very occasionally, there is an excessively high and dense block, indicated by significant numbness, especially if above the nipples. The combination of a high block and hypotension is the one indication to turn off the epidural infusion, and may require treatment with ephedrine (3–6 mg i.v., repeated at 5-min intervals). Involve an anaesthetist.

3. *Pruritus (itching).* This can be extremely troubling. Try an antihistamine first, for example chorpheniramine 10–20 mg i.m. If this is ineffective, reduce the rate of infusion, and give a *small* dose of naloxone (e.g. 0.1 mg i.v.).

4. *Urinary retention.* This is common. Patients are usually catheterized. This can limit the usefulness of epidural analgesia in orthopaedic implant surgery, because catheterization leads to an increase in implant infection rate. (This might not be so if suprapubic catheters were used routinely, but that's another story.)

5. *Drug errors.* All manner of drugs get put down the epidural by mistake from time to time, but few cause real harm (phenol, neat potassium chloride and alcohol are exceptions). More worrying is when someone gives a local anaesthetic infusion intravenously. This can lead to local anaesthetic toxicity (see below).

    Air in the epidural space is harmless.

6. *Nausea.* This is usually as a result of the opioid, but occasionally is due to hypotension.

7. *Sedation.* By and large, epidural infusions do not cause sedation, but when they do it may be a sign of impending respiratory depression (along with pupil constriction). Reduce the infusion rate, but look for another cause of drowsiness.

8. *Motor or sensory block.* Patients commonly come back from theatre with persistent motor or sensory block, resulting from the use of concentrated local anaesthetic during the procedure. It can be a source of distress, but reassurance that sensation will slowly return may be enough.

    The extremely rare complication of epidural haematoma causing cord compression results in severe back pain, and a *spastic* (rather than flaccid) paralysis of the lower limbs. The patient needs urgent referral to a neurosurgeon, as the haematoma must be evacuated within 6 h to have a chance of avoiding permanent paralysis.

9. *Headache.* This can occur after a **dural tap**, which occurs in about 1% of epidurals. During the insertion of the epidural, the dura and arachnoid meninges sometimes get punctured accidentally. This allows a leak of CSF out into the epidural space and the fall in CSF pressure or volume leads to a 'spinal headache'. This is like the world's worst hangover. The pain may be in the neck, occiput or frontal region. The main point in the history is that the pain is postural, and usually disappears completely on lying flat. You are going to need expert help in dealing with this problem;

refer it to an anaesthetist. However, you can help by ensuring good general hydration (so that the manufacture of more CSF can continue) and preventing constipation (straining at stool temporarily increases CSF pressure, thus encouraging more leakage). Spinal headache is not an indication to stop the epidural.

10. *Local anaesthetic toxicity.* This is immensely rare, but it can happen if an infusion is given intravenously by accident. The organ most affected is the brain. Early signs include restlessness, agitation, tinnitus, circumoral tingling or numbness and, in severe cases, convulsions and coma. Cardiovascular manifestations are usually secondary to CNS toxicity, although bupivacaine overdose is associated with a resistant form of ventricular tachycardia. The most important job is to spot the early signs and stop further local anaesthetic infusion. Get advice from an anaesthetist.

Analgesia in difficult circumstances

Pain teams exist to help in any awkward situation.

Respiratory disease
This can be tricky, but it is one situation where pain is definitely more dangerous than analgesia. This is covered in Chapter II.17.

CNS depression
Sometimes, a conscious patient with a head injury is in severe pain. Since the observation of such a patient is crucially dependent upon changes in conscious level, sedative drugs (e.g. opioids) might be thought to be undesirable. This concern has led to codeine being the drug most commonly prescribed. As I mentioned earlier, this is dodging the issue. If codeine doesn't alter conscious level, it's because it doesn't provide useful analgesia. You may as well not bother.

Codeine preparations are a good choice for mild to moderate pain. Severe pain is in fact very bad for the injured brain, and cannot be ignored. If there is conflict between analgesia and monitoring, the patient may need to be nursed in a higher dependency area (e.g. HDU or ITU). Patient-controlled analgesia is entirely appropriate for pain management in this situation. Avoid using papaveretum, which is a bit more sedating than the others.

Shock
The treatment of acute pain in the presence of shock is extremely hazardous, and the decision to give opioids should be left to someone senior. This most commonly happens after major trauma, where the patient is suffering acute pain despite severe hypovolaemia. As a general rule, shock should be treated as far as possible before analgesia is given.

If analgesics are considered necessary, a good drug to use is i.v. fentanyl in increments of 25–50 mcg. This has the advantage of being short-acting and having a relatively neutral effect on the cardiovascular system. Never, **never** give i.m. drugs of *any* kind to a shocked patient.

Narcotic addiction
The management of surgical pain in drug addicts is complex and ungratifying.

For our purposes, such patients can be divided into three groups:

1. *The true addict*. His life is ruled by his need for narcotics. What he fears most in the world is withdrawal. These patients usually present as emergencies, most often after trauma.
2. *The recreational user*. This person takes a bit of this and a bit of that, but may not fear withdrawal as much. These patients are the most difficult to manage.
3. *The reformed user*. He has been clean for a while and is very keen to avoid having to take opioids. Not an addict at all, really. His wishes should be followed if at all possible, and you should engage the help of an acute pain specialist.

You have two jobs: provide analgesia and prevent withdrawal. You are not running the Betty Ford clinic.

Some otherwise reputable texts advise us to avoid giving opioids to drug users. This is utterly futile. Like it or not, you are going to have give these patients what they want: morphine. Rid yourself of high-minded ideas of getting the patient off drugs. The period immediately after they were run over by a bus is not the best time. Epidurals, nerve blocks and such like are never the whole answer, because they do nothing to prevent withdrawal. Get advice from a specialist in substance abuse right at the start.

The true addict may actually be easy to manage if you gain his trust. The simple way to do this is to promise him that you won't let him go into withdrawal, and that you will believe him when he complains of pain. Patient-controlled analgesia is not necessarily contraindicated, and allows daily opioid requirements to be measured. This may seem daft, and is controversial, but there is evidence from America to show that although drug users have a higher dose requirement (~50 mg morphine per day higher on average), they do not stay on a pump any longer than non-addicts. As the patient recovers, you can start weaning, with the guidance of an expert in substance abuse.

Children

The average houseman will not be looking after children having major surgery, but there are certain problems associated with pain management in kids.

- Although many children will vocally demonstrate the presence of pain, many respond by withdrawing. Pain assessment is thus difficult.
- Intramuscular analgesia is especially problematic in children, although a single dose is acceptable.
- Patient-controlled analgesia has been used successfully in children, down to the age of 5, though for smaller children this requires specialized supervision. Epidurals and continuous i.v. infusions can also be used.
- Most mild to moderate pain can be managed with a combination of local anaesthesia to the wound, paracetamol or voltarol suppository, regular oral medication (with elixirs), and 'rescue' opioids (e.g. 1 mg/kg pethidine or 200 mcg/kg of morphine).

Neurogenic pain

Neurogenic pain can occur as a result of nerve injury or spontaneously. It is a far too complex topic to cover in detail, but you ought to be able to pick out patients who may benefit from specialist referral.

In a nutshell:

- Neurogenic pain is striking for the fact that it does not respond to opioids. If a patient is still in pain despite large doses of opioid, don't immediately label them as malingerers, as this is one of the factors responsible for the paranoid 'chronic pain personality'.
- Neurogenic pain is often 'lancinating' (shooting or electric) and may be triggered by touching a certain spot. Pain may also result from stimuli that are not normally painful.

Treatment should be carried out by a specialist, but may involve drugs that are not normally considered analgesics (carbamazepine, amytriptyline, baclofen), nerve blocks or neurosurgery.

Chapter II.5

NAUSEA AND VOMITING

Chapter II.5

NAUSEA AND VOMITING

KEY POINTS

The causes of perioperative nausea and vomiting (PONV) are complex. Very rarely is it 'just the anaesthetic'.

Nausea and vomiting cause fluid loss, myocardial strain, oesophageal rupture and cost money.

Prochlorperazine is the first line drug of choice.

Metoclopramide quite simply **does not work** for PONV.

In refractory cases, droperidol, cyclizine, hyoscine, ondansetron and acupuncture are all worth a try.

Droperidol, metoclopramide, prochlorperazine, haloperidol and chlorpromazine are all **antidopaminergic**. This means they can cause extrapyramidal side-effects. Acute dystonia can be treated with procyclidine 5 mg i.m.

Exclude other causes of persistent vomiting. Keep a close eye on fluid and electrolyte requirements.

Physiology of emesis

Vomiting is essentially a reflex, consisting of emetic detectors, a central integrating area and motor outputs.

There are four main emetic detectors:
1. The chemoreceptor trigger zone
2. The vestibular system
3. Gastrointestinal afferents
4. Higher centres.

Why do patients vomit after surgery?
Well, I'm glad you asked that. There are a large number of factors involved.

Preoperative factors
Many patients presenting for surgery have conditions which themselves are potent causes of nausea and vomiting, for example raised intracranial pressure or bowel obstruction. Even when surgery alleviates the condition, PONV is more common in these patients, suggesting that the emetic reflexes have been sensitized. Surgery in the presence of a full stomach, as in emergency procedures, or following trauma when gastric emptying is greatly slowed, carries a higher incidence of vomiting, as does surgery in the presence of alcohol. (In the *patient*, I mean.)

Direct drug actions

Opioid receptors are present on the cells of the chemoreceptor trigger zone, and all opioid agonists exert a dose-dependent emetic effect. They also cause delayed gastric emptying, sensitize the emetic response to labyrinthine stimuli and enhance the release of 5-hydroxytryptamine (5-HT) from the gut.

Not much else is known about the direct effects of anaesthetic drugs on the vomiting reflex. Some agents are worse than others, but no mechanisms to explain the differences are known, and it is extremely difficult to separate the various factors at play. Propofol, an increasingly popular anaesthetic agent, is an anti-emetic.

Indirect drug effects

- *Gastrointestinal effects:* many anaesthetic agents reduce gut motility, and some inhalational agents, particularly nitrous oxide, may diffuse into the gut lumen causing distension.
- *Cardiovascular effects:* hypotension, particularly that which is associated with spinal anaesthesia, may lead to nausea and vomiting.
- *CNS effects:* drug-induced rises in intracranial pressure may worsen nausea. Also, diffusion of gases into the middle ear has been suggested as a cause.

Patient factors

After all this talk about the esoteric actions of various drugs, it ought to be mentioned that certain patients are going to throw up no matter *what* you do.

- *Age:* the incidence of PONV peaks at early adolescence, and then stays constant throughout adult life, declining slightly in the elderly.
- *Motion sickness:* patients who suffer from motion sickness are significantly more likely to suffer from PONV.
- *Previous PONV:* nausea and vomiting is considerably (up to three times) more common in patients with prior history of PONV, whatever the cause. Such patients are also, anecdotally, harder to treat. The theory is that this is an example of 'learned aversion', a powerful defensive mechanism, that makes sure you never ever forget what it was that made you sick, to prevent you ingesting it again (unless it was beer).
- *Sex:* the incidence of PONV in adult females is approximately two to three times that in adult males. PONV is significantly higher if surgery is carried out in the third and fourth weeks of the menstrual cycle.
- *Anxiety:* possible mechanisms are inadvertent swallowing of air (aerophagy) and delayed gastric emptying.
- *Obesity.*

Effects of the surgical procedure

- *Site of surgery:* some operations are more strongly associated with PONV than others. For example, intra-abdominal surgery carries an incidence of about 70%, compared with 15% for abdominal wall surgery. Laparoscopic gynae surgery, ear surgery, surgery for correction of squint and adenotonsillectomy all carry a high incidence. Low incidences are found after dental surgery, D&C and surgery to the extremities.
- *Duration of surgery:* the longer the surgery, the higher the incidence.
- *Pain:* unrelieved pain has been shown to be a cause in itself of PONV. In this situation, the use of opioids can actually relieve nausea.

Surgical complications
Finally, don't forget that some important complications occurring in the postoperative period may present with nausea and vomiting. Ileus, bowel obstruction and pancreatitis spring to mind.

Complications of nausea and vomiting

- *Fluid and electrolyte loss*: fluid deficits can be large, and are commonly seen in patients who stuck it out a bit too long at home before presenting with their acute surgical abdomen. Electrolyte disturbances, such as hypokalaemia or alkalosis, are also common.
- *Physical effects*: violent retching and vomiting can lead to wound dehiscence and bleeding from suture lines, haematemesis from a Mallory–Wiess tear to the distal oesophagus, worsening of pain from abdominal wounds and, rarely, oesophageal rupture. The latter is particularly dangerous, and can lead to fatal mediastinitis if not treated.
- *Physiological effects*: vomiting is accompanied by hypertension and tachycardia, which may have serious consequences, particularly in the elderly and arteriopathic populations. Myocardial infarction, cerebrovascular events and damage to vein grafts, particularly after cardiac surgery, may all occur.
- *Financial effects*: on top of all this, PONV is actually quite expensive, particularly if it occurs after day-case surgery, and the patient has to be admitted.

Treatments and prevention

The measures currently available to treat PONV are certainly not perfect. However, there is no doubt that most patients do not even receive the full benefits of the measures available.

General measures
The most important non-pharmacological manoeuvre is placement of a nasogastric tube. This will reduce the incidence of nausea and vomiting in those with non-functioning guts, and allows monitoring of the return of gut function. Some people claim relief from elasticated wrist bands ('sea bands'). Conventional acupuncture, when administered at the P6 point in the wrist, has been shown in several studies to be at least as effective as prochlor-perazine, and this technique may well become more widely used. For the time being, however, the mainstay of treatment is with drugs.

The drugs used to treat nausea and vomiting fall into six main categories, as summarized opposite.

Phenothiazines
These are the most useful agents for treatment of PONV. They act by blocking dopamine receptors on the chemoreceptor trigger zone. Prochlorperazine is the most commonly used agent in this group, and it works. A 73% reduction in PONV has been demonstrated after gynae laparoscopy.

Prochlorperazine is available via the oral, rectal and i.m. routes. Elimination half-life is 6.8 h, and the usual i.m. dose for an adult is 12.5 mg 8-hourly.

Class of drug	Examples
Phenothiazines	Prochlorperazine (Stemetil®)
Butyrophenones	Droperidol Haloperidol
Anticholinergics	Hyoscine (Scopolamine®)
GI prokinetic drugs	Metoclopramide (Maxolon®) Domperidone
Antihistamines	Cyclizine (Valoid®)
5-HT$_3$ antagonists	Ondansetron

The most important adverse reactions to these drugs are **extrapyramidal side-effects (EPSEs)**. These are a consequence of their antidopaminergic action, which can induce a Parkinsonian-like state. Acute dystonias affect the face and neck, leading to uncontrollable lip-smacking and other bizarre actions. They are extremely unpleasant. The incidence has been estimated at 0.3% of those receiving prochlorperazine. It is extremely uncommon after doses of <10 mg. Most at risk are children, and young women. EPSEs can be rapidly treated with **procyclidine**, a centrally acting anticholinergic agent. The usual dose is 5 mg i.m.

Other side effects, common to all phenothiazines, include sedation, hypotension, cholestatic jaundice, skin sensitivity and hyperprolactinaemia.

Butyrophenones
Haloperidol, an important antipsychotic, is a prominent member of this group, but it is only droperidol which is used for treatment of PONV. Many studies have confirmed the efficacy of droperidol, but the effect is less striking than prochlorperazine. EPSEs occur rarely after droperidol (it too, is antidopaminergic), but may happen after small doses, and have delayed onset. Hypotension can also occur due to α-blockade.

In addition, about 20% of patients who receive droperidol complain later of an extremely unpleasant feeling of malaise and anxiety, which they feel completely unable to convey at the time. Indeed, anyone given a big enough dose takes on a rather vacant appearance, and it comes as no surprise that related compounds are used to get people to behave themselves.

Anticholinergics
Most commonly used is hyoscine, which for years was the standard premedicant [along with papaveretum (Omnopon)]. The usual dose is 0.2–0.3 mg i.m. for the average adult, and its half-life is approximately 2 h. Sedation and typical anticholinergic effects, such as dry mouth and blurring of vision, are the commonest side effects. Psychosis may occur in the elderly. Hyoscine can also be given as a transdermal preparation, which has been widely used in motion sickness. A couple of studies have shown it to be effective when applied a few hours before surgery. This may be worth thinking about for the frequent nausea sufferer.

GI prokinetic drugs

The most common member of this group, and probably the most frequently prescribed anti-emetic of all, is *metoclopramide* ('Maxolon').

Metoclopramide acts both by increasing the motility of the GI tract, and by blocking dopamine receptors at the chemoreceptor trigger zone. It has also been shown to block 5-HT$_3$ receptors at the CTZ, which may explain its effect in high dose during chemotherapy. The popularity of this agent is in part due to this attractive 'dual action' concept, and the availability of an i.v. preparation.

There is only one problem, which may come as a surprise to fans of metoclopramide: it doesn't work.

In over **half** the studies carried out on metoclopramide, it was no better than placebo. In several comparative studies, metoclopramide was consistently shown to be four to five times less effective than droperidol. Although there are situations in which it may be useful, there seems to be no justification for using metoclopramide as first line treatment or prevention in PONV.

EPSEs occur with metoclopramide. Cardiovascular problems have been reported with i.v. administration. The usual dose is 10 mg i.v., i.m. or orally. Plasma half-life is 4 h, which is significantly shorter than other anti-emetic drugs.

Domperidone was developed in order not to cross the blood–brain barrier, in an attempt to prevent EPSEs. The parenteral preparation was withdrawn fairly quickly after reports of dysrhythmias, and it is now given only rectally. There is little evidence to support its effectiveness, and it is little used in PONV.

Antihistamines

Cyclizine is the only drug in this group used in PONV. It has both antihistamine and anticholinergic actions, and is effective in both prevention and treatment. It is not a dopamine antagonist, and therefore does not cause EPSEs. Side-effects are mild, dry mouth, visual disturbances and light sedation being the most common. It may be given i.v., i.m., orally and subcutaneously. An infusion given subcutaneously (150 mg over 24 h) is particularly effective. It is often prescribed as a compound preparation with morphine (Cyclimorph®), especially in general practice.

It is a drug which is often overlooked, but can be extremely useful, especially in refractory cases.

Ondansetron

Ondansetron is a 5-HT$_3$ antagonist, designed specifically for the job. It was used originally, with spectacular success, for the nausea and vomiting of chemotherapy. A sales drive is currently under way to persuade us to use it in PONV. Although it shows considerable promise, and has a low incidence of side-effects, its high cost and the lack of comparative data make it an agent to be used only in specific circumstances, when other methods have failed, or for prophylaxis in high risk cases.

Chapter II.6

FLUID AND ELECTROLYTE BALANCE

Chapter II.6

FLUID AND ELECTROLYTE BALANCE

KEY POINTS

If what comes out is put back in, a stable patient will remain stable. The difficulty is knowing what has come out.

Normal maintenance requirements are 30 ml/kg/day of water, 1–2 mmol/kg/day of sodium and 1 mmol/kg/day of potassium. Note this is about 2 l/day for an average adult.

Replacing fluid loss is an inexact science, assessment is difficult. Fluid charts are useful, but do not tell the whole story.

Avoid the 'houseman's regimen'. Use combinations of normal saline and 5% dextrose for maintenance.

Patients who are stressed (e.g. after major surgery) **cannot handle large water loads**. Excessive use of 5% dextrose or dextrose–saline can lead to hyponatraemia and pulmonary oedema.

Patients with cardiac failure have the same maintenance fluid requirements as everyone else. A history of cardiac failure is not a guarantee against hypovolaemia.

Introduction

Most doctors qualify without anyone telling them, in practical terms, what fluids to give a surgical patient and why. What little we are taught is usually wrong. As a result, a wide range of errors is seen in the prescription of perioperative fluids.

It may seem that few problems occur as a result, but it is known, for example, that overhydration makes the lungs stiffer, impairs gas exchange, causes peripheral oedema, inhibits wound healing, and may even contribute to multiple organ failure. Underhydration causes renal and cardiovascular damage, and carries a significant mortality. All these effects are worse in patients with chronic disease.

Physiology

This, we have pruned to its bare essentials:

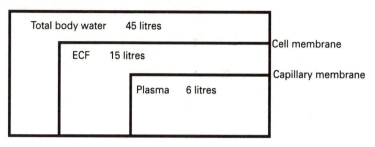

Electrolyte contents (mmol/l)

	Sodium	Potassium
Intracellular	15	150
Extracellular	145	4.5

Figure II.6.1.   Normal fluid volumes and electrolyte contents. Notice that most of your potassium is intracellular, while most of your sodium is extracellular.

Normal maintenance requirements
Normal maintenance is the fluid required to replace the *normal* losses. If you remember nothing else, remember these three numbers:
- Water: 30 ml/kg/day
- Sodium: 1–2 mmol/kg/day
- Potassium: 1 mmol/kg/day

Deficits and losses

Normal losses
Fluid is lost under normal circumstances as urine, and as 'insensible losses'. Urine output is variable, but an average figure is about 1500 ml/day for a 70 kg adult. Insensible losses are accounted for mainly by sweat, with smaller losses from secretions, faeces, etc. Under normal circumstances, insensible loss is approximately 0.5 ml/kg/h, though this figure can vary wildly. Fever, obesity and high environmental temperature all lead to increased insensible loss, sometimes up to 3 l/day.

Special surgical losses
Blood loss. Blood loss in theatre is usually recorded in the notes, or rather an estimate of blood loss is. Figures for blood loss are notoriously inaccurate, even when meticulous attention is paid to it, for example by weighing swabs. Blood loss may also be occult, for example retroperitoneal haematoma in pelvic fracture.

'Third space losses'. Injury of any kind causes an increase in local capillary permeability which allows fluid to leak into the interstitial space. This fluid is lost to the circulation despite remaining within the body. Sequestration of fluids may occur in inflamed wounds, the peritoneal cavity in peritonitis and into diluted loops of bowel during an ileus. There is debate as to the significance of third space fluid loss in the majority of patients, but in the case of bowel obstruction or crush injury such losses can be huge. It is important to note, however, that upon convalescence and healing, much of this sequestered fluid will be reclaimed by the circulation.

Other measured losses. Any significant volumes of fluid retrieved from nasogastric tubes, vomit, diarrhoea, bile, etc., should be recorded and taken into consideration. Remember also that these secretions are rich in electrolytes which also need to be replaced:

Fluid	Na (mmol/l)	K (mmol/l)	Cl (mmol/l)	HCO_3 (mmol/l)
Gastric	50	15	140	0–15
Pancreatic	130	5	55	110
Bile	145	5	100	38
Ileal	140	11	70	variable
Diarrhoea	30–140	**30–70**	–	**20–80**

Notice in particular the huge potassium losses that can occur with diarrhoea.

Pre-existing deficits

This is probably the most difficult element of fluid balance to estimate. Very few patients keep a fluid balance chart at home, and it is almost impossible to judge how much fluid is lost through vomiting or diarrhoea. Blood loss out of hospital is also hard to estimate. It may be overestimated, as even a small amount of blood can look pretty dramatic, or underestimated, as in scalp lacerations that can bleed a surprising amount. The only way is to simply be aware of the situations in which a patient may present with large deficits (i.e. bowel obstruction, prolonged vomiting, diarrhoea).

Other deficits are iatrogenic. 'Nil by mouth from midnight' can give rise to significant deficits by the time surgery is performed, especially in children. Osmotic purgatives used in bowel prep can do the same.

Stress and fluid balance

The stress response affects fluid balance in a way which deserves a special mention. Anyone subjected to injury from trauma or surgery exhibits some form of stress response. As part of that response, the hormones aldosterone and ADH are secreted in large amounts, which results in salt and water retention. This has led some to the terrifying conclusion that stressed patients do not require any sodium, and are best managed with 3 l of 5% dextrose per day. This is gross oversimplification and dangerous practice. If you give this to your patients they will drown.

There is indeed sodium and water retention after major surgery, and occasionally this leads to oliguria. Sodium reabsorption is increased by a variety of mechanisms, by the action of aldosterone on the distal tubule, but much more importantly by a variety of effects causing increased reabsorption in the *proximal* tubule. Increased absorption in the proximal tubule leads to less solute being delivered to the ascending loop of Henle. This is the only part where sodium is absorbed without water, and it results in an inability to make dilute urine. This effect is greatly exaggerated at times of stress because of the great increase in secretion of ADH. Stressed patients therefore **cannot excrete large water loads**.

Appropriate fluid therapy can modify the salt retention, reduce the levels of hormones like renin and angiotensin, and prevent oliguria. It does not appear to be possible to modify the dramatic increase in ADH secretion, and thus use of hypotonic solutions will lead to water retention, with hyponatraemia and pulmonary oedema.

The other point is that although the healthy kidneys avidly retain sodium after major surgery, sodium is being lost elsewhere, into 'third spaces' and as blood or gastrointestinal losses. Also, the diseased kidney cannot retain sodium as avidly in conditions of deprivation, and it has been estimated that 50% of elderly patients presenting for surgery have renal salt-losing state.

Management

I.v. fluids
Ignoring blood products, there are two basic classes of i.v. fluids: crystalloid, which contain only small particles such as sodium and chloride ions or glucose, and colloids which all contain larger molecules capable of exerting oncotic pressure.

Crystalloids. Fluid shifts between ICF and ECF occur by osmosis. Since sodium is the most osmotically important ion, the distribution of a given volume of i.v. fluid within the body depends primarily on its sodium content. Thus, the available fluids fall into three groups:
1. Normal (0.9%) saline and Hartmann's solution (Ringer's lactate) contain 150 mmol/l (or thereabouts) of sodium, similar to extracellular fluid. These solutions will be distributed in the extracellular fluid compartment.
2. 5% Dextrose. All the sugar in this solution gets rapidly pulled into cells and burnt or made into glycogen, so giving 5% dextrose is essentially giving pure water. It will distribute itself throughout the total body water.
3. 'Dextrose/saline' falls between the two. It has some sodium, so a proportion of the water (20%) stays in the ECF, but the majority ends up in total body water.

Colloids. Colloids are solutions that contain molecules of one sort or another that are too big to pass across capillary membranes. Under normal circumstances, such fluids are retained within the intravascular space, useful if rapid intravascular expansion is required. The most commonly used colloids are the gelatins, Haemaccel and Gelofusine, which are made from cows. Others include Hetastarch and the dextrans, and naturally occurring colloids such as albumin, and fresh frozen plasma.

Although colloid solutions have attractive advantages in some situations, there are important drawbacks. They are very much more expensive than crystalloid solutions, and there is a significant incidence of anaphylaxis. Although in normal circumstances colloid solutions are retained in the intravascular space, shock and injury (the sort of conditions where they are most often used) can lead to an increase in capillary permeability, thus allowing smaller colloid molecules to reach the interstitial space, where they will act to draw fluid out into the tissues, worsening oedema. This is the basis of the 'colloid vs. crystalloid' argument that has raged for a number of years. Albumin is probably the 'best' colloid, but is too expensive for routine use.

Assessment

Decisions on fluid management should follow the usual process of clinical assessment. Unfortunately, the best available clinical indicators are only crude methods of detecting fluid balance abnormalities.

Nevertheless, assessment should include:

- History: ask specifically about thirst, prolonged vomiting and diarrhoea, any out-of-hospital blood losses. Note if the surgical problem is one normally associated with large fluid deficits, for example bowel obstruction, crush injury, pelvic fracture, pancreatitis. Some of the symptoms of underreplacement are subtle: drowsiness, headaches, dizziness, malaise and delayed mobilization.
- Fluid balance chart: this is a vitally important document, particularly in the postoperative period when input and output get complicated. Accurate information about all measurable fluid gains and losses is usually available. It is very important, however, that it is considered bearing in mind the information that it *doesn't* give you: prior deficits, insensible loss, third space loss, internal haemorrhage.
- Clinical examination: look for dry mucous membranes, oedema, pulse rate and pressure, warm/cold peripheries, basal crepitations, skin turgor (unreliable in the elderly). Daily weights are a sensitive measure of overall fluid balance. Examination may only detect gross abnormalities, for example skin turgor is only changed after a 5% drop in body weight. Note also that oedema and hypovolaemia are not mutually exclusive.
- Urine output: a urine volume of 0.5–1 ml/kg/h is acceptable. Oliguria is most commonly caused by inadequate volume, but renal impairment and urinary obstruction must be excluded (see Chapter II.18).
- CVP: serial measurements of CVP are useful in fluid assessment. However, individual measurements can be misleading (see Chapter II.11).
- Haematology: haemoglobin and haematocrit may point to unexpected blood loss. Acute haemorrhage may not be reflected in lab values for several hours, however.
- Biochemistry: urea rises in dehydration, and in severe cases so does sodium.
- Chest X-ray: can demonstrate 'wet lungs' (see Chapter II.17), thus pointing to overhydration. This is useful in highly complex ITU situations, but it is not for routine assessment of fluid balance.

Planning a regimen

Despite the difficulties that can occur, the majority of surgical patients will have uncomplicated and predictable fluid requirements after surgery. The aim is to produce a stable but *slightly* dry patient. For any patient, the equation is the same:

> fluid required =
> pre-existing deficit + normal maintenance + ongoing losses.

You should plan your regimen so as to address each of the three parts of the equation separately. As we have seen, knowing these figures with accuracy is difficult. Current experience suggests that we tend to overestimate the 'maintenance' part, but grossly underestimate the 'pre-existing deficit' part.

First of all, for goodness' sake avoid the 'houseman's regimen', that is 3000 ml of dextrose–saline a day in every patient. There are very few patients for whom this is an appropriate regimen. This gives you either too little sodium, or too much water, or both.

Pre-existing deficit. If you think your patient has a pre-existing deficit, treat it **there and then**, with a fluid challenge servo loop. Give a fluid bolus (e.g. 250 ml saline stat), reassess haemodynamic status and urine output, repeat until you think the patient is filled. It makes no sense to just 'speed up the drip' and leave.

Maintenance. Remember the daily maintenance requirements: 30 ml/kg of water, 1–2 mmol/kg of sodium. For a 70 kg adult, this works out as about 2000 ml of water with about 70–140 mmol of sodium. Hence, for stable patient with minimal ongoing losses (e.g. after cholecystectomy) **500 ml of 0.9% saline plus 1500 ml of 5% dextrose over 24 h** is plenty. Most patients who receive more than 1500 ml of 5% dextrose per day become hyponatraemic.

Ongoing losses. If the patient has ongoing losses, they are likely to be sodium-containing ones, so any fluid additional to the above should be given as normal saline or Hartmann's. So, for more major surgery, for example colonic resections, aneurysm repair, thoracotomy **1.5–2.0 l of 5% dextrose plus 1000 ml of 0.9% saline over 24 h** is suitable. In addition to this salt and water therapy, the patient will need:

- Potassium. After the first day, the patient should receive 1 mmol/kg/day somehow. If still totally reliant on parenteral fluids this should be given as 20–40 mmol KCl in each litre bag.
- Blood, as required to maintain haemoglobin above 10 g/dl.
- Replacement for measured gastrointestinal losses (e.g. nasogastric aspirates, biliary drainage). This is best achieved by giving an equivalent volume of saline with 20 mmol/l KCl. Large losses should have electrolyte content measured to ensure appropriate replacement.
- Nutrition. If fluid therapy is continued beyond the third postoperative day, then artificial feeding should be considered (see Chapter II.8). Note that low plasma albumin is a sign of poor nutritional state, and will not respond to optimistic attempts at replacement with expensive albumin solutions.
- **Daily U&Es whilst on i.v. fluids**.

Special situations

Rule number one: if what comes out (water, sodium, potassium, red cells) is put back, a stable patient will remain stable.

This is sometimes easier said than done but it is the principle which should govern fluid management in any unusual situation.

Cardiac failure

There is a generalized tendency, encouraged by some otherwise reputable textbooks, to reduce or even halve the maintenance fluid for patients with a history of heart failure. Heart failure does not affect the rate of fluid loss, and restricting intake is daft. *Maintenance* fluid and electrolyte requirements are the **same**.

The difference is that those with myocardial dysfunction cannot cope with as wide a range of filling pressure (high or low) as healthy individuals, so aggressive fluid resuscitation should only be used when there is good evidence of ECF loss or deficit. Diuretics should be continued, to prevent excessive sodium retention.

Clinical signs of fluid status are even more unreliable than usual, though *changes* in physical signs are important. Serial CVP measurements are useful, but don't expect the values for CVP necessarily to be in the 'normal range'. Daily weights are extremely useful for monitoring day-to-day fluid balance. Remember that patients with cardiac failure may still become hypovolaemic, and become very ill when they do. The normal process of fluid challenge should be employed (albeit slightly more cautiously) as first line treatment in the event of hypotension or oliguria.

Respiratory disease

When treating patients with chronic lung disease, the tightrope is narrower than usual. Small and clinically undetectable degrees of fluid overload can dramatically worsen lung function, and it is probably better to err on the dry side. However, dehydration makes sputum more tenacious and harder to clear. Patients in respiratory distress have higher insensible losses, though this effect can be lessened with the use of humidifed oxygen. CVP readings will be higher than expected, but this does not necessarily imply fluid overload.

Liver disease

Patients with obstructive jaundice are at risk of perioperative renal failure (the hepatorenal syndrome), which is best prevented by maintaining a high urine output, either with greater than usual maintenance fluid, or osmotic diuretics such as mannitol, or both.

Patients with liver disease are only really a fluid balance problem where there is ascites, and such patients are uncommon outside specialized units, thankfully. The key to success is maintaining a zero sodium balance, as excessive sodium intake will expand the ascitic fluid. Serum sodium is often low, but total body sodium stores are raised. In the absence of other losses, 50 mmol of sodium per day is adequate. Patients with varices are at risk of occult gastrointestinal haemorrhage.

Renal disease

Patients with chronic renal failure who are on dialysis pose considerable fluid management problems in the perioperative period, but they are usually managed by renal physicians or ITU postoperatively. Of more concern to the average house officer are patients with 'renal impairment'. This can mean anything from clinically undetectable kidney disease to those teetering on the brink of long-term dialysis. For patients already under the care of a renal physician, the unit should be contacted for advice, or even for transfer. For the others, a few general points:

- Strict fluid balance records should be kept, U&Es should be done daily. CVP monitoring is useful, especially for major surgery. Hourly urine output measurements are mandatory.
- It is probably best, as a rule, to err on the wet side. This is because nothing will finish off a failing kidney quicker than hypovolaemia. Bear in mind, though, that many such patients have reduced ability to handle large water or sodium loads, so don't go mad.
- Avoid potentially nephrotoxic drugs unless OK'd by a renal physician: NSAIDs, aminoglycosides, loop diuretics.

Patients at risk of renal problems postoperatively are the elderly, those on long-term NSAIDs, those with severe atherosclerosis, diabetics, and anyone with a raised preoperative creatinine level. More advice on management of renal failure is available in Chapter II.18.

Diabetics
Diabetic control often goes awry as a result of acute surgical illness and, if glucose levels have been elevated for a while, the patient may be severely dehydrated on presentation. The fluid management of diabetics presenting for elective surgery need not be any different, but bear in mind that renal impairment is not uncommon in this population. For more on preparation of the diabetic, see Chapter I.7.

Other problems
Septic shock. This is generalized sepsis that leads to vasodilation and hypotension. In its early stages, progressive vasodilation causes relative hypovolaemia, and fluid resuscitation is required to restore blood pressure. Often huge volumes are required, which will often worry people who enjoy looking at fluid balance charts and declaring a patient to be overloaded.

Hypothermia. Repeated bolus fluid resuscitation may be required as a hypothermic patient warms up, and previously unperfused peripheral vascular beds are reopened. Again, don't start fretting about 'positive balance' if the patient is clinically well.

Hormone problems. Hormone problems may occur, such as diabetes insipidus and Addison's disease. Seek help from an endocrinologist *before* surgery.

Electrolyte disturbances

Hypokalaemia
The definition of hypokalaemia is serum potassium <3.5 mmol/l (though levels >3.0 are tolerable) Severe hypokalaemia produces striking symptoms of muscle weakness.

Causes include excessive K^+ loss (diarrhoea, vomiting) or inadequate replacement, alkalosis, diuretic therapy, bicarbonate, glucose–insulin, salbutamol, hyperventilation, tricyclic overdose.

For management of hypokalaemia, the average adult needs 60 mmol/day maintenance. Correction of defects will require more. Oral is best if possible, for example Slow K three tabs 6-hourly. If giving it i.v., 40 mmol is about the most you can get into a litre of fluid safely.

Hyperkalaemia

Acute hyperkalaemia is an emergency. It is defined as serum potassium >5.0 mmol/l. Start getting scared when it's 6.0 or more. Acute changes are much more dangerous than chronic changes.

It may be caused by renal failure, acidosis from any cause, potassium-sparing diuretics given with potassium supplements, hypercatabolism, for example malignant hyperthermia.

For management of hyperkalaemia:

1. 10 ml of 10% calcium gluconate i.v. slowly. This protects the myocardium from the dysrhythmic effects of hyperkalaemia, for about half an hour.
2. If there is acidosis (there usually is), correct it. The formula:

$$\text{base deficit} \times \text{body weight (kg)} \times 0.3$$

   gives the total volume of 8.4% bicarbonate (in ml) required. Give half this amount initially.
3. Give dextrose and insulin, for example 50 ml of 50% dextrose with 20 units of soluble insulin over 30 min.

None of these measures removes potassium from the body. To do this either:

4. Give calcium resonium 30 g t.i.d. orally or rectally, or
5. Arrange dialysis, for acute renal failure.

Hyponatraemia

Abnormalities in sodium concentration are much more commonly caused by changes in levels of *solvent* (i.e. water) than of solute.

Hyponatraemia is therefore usually a sign of excessive water. The commonest cause is iatrogenic, that is following excessive use of 5% dextrose or dextrose–saline. The other important cause is TUR syndrome, a potentially fatal complication of transurethral resection of prostate (see Chapter II.22). The syndrome of inappropriate ADH secretion leads to excessive retention of water and occurs with some lung tumours and CNS lesions. Excessive treatment with oxytocin during labour can cause hyponatraemia, as it has a significant ADH-like effect.

Excessive sodium-rich fluid losses can lead to hyponatraemia, although serum sodium more frequently remains unchanged. The commonest cause of chronic hyponatraemia is long-term diuretic therapy.

The critical decision to make in the management of hyponatraemia is whether there is overhydration or underhydration. This may be more easily judged by the history than clinical examination, unless there is a gross abnormality.

For *acute dilutional hyponatraemia* the approach should be water restriction. Saline may be given if there are ongoing sodium losses. Omit 5% dextrose or dextrose–saline from the fluid regimen. **TUR syndrome** is a special case, and is considered in Chapter II.22.

Acute salt-losing hyponatraemia should be tackled by resuscitation with 0.9% saline and appropriate potassium. Correction of hypovolaemia allows restoration of salt–water balance.

Diuretic-induced hyponatraemia can be treated by discontinuation of the offending drug, though this may take some time. It may be undesirable to correct too quickly.

Use of hypertonic saline solutions can be extremely hazardous, especially where the patient is already overloaded. Their use should be restricted to severe, acute hyponatraemia associated with hypovolaemia. Even then they should be used with extreme caution.

Hypernatraemia

This is nearly always a sign of true dehydration, that is lack of water. The hypovolaemia is usually clinically obvious. Although the lack of water is severe, there is usually a total body sodium deficit as well. Fluid resuscitation with 5% dextrose or dextrose–saline is the usual answer.

Chapter II.7

BLEEDING AND TRANFUSION

Chapter II.7

BLEEDING AND TRANSFUSION

KEY POINTS

The volume lost is estimated by charting vital signs, which also guide fluid resuscitation. Tachycardia is an early sign; hypotension only occurs late. Urine output and conscious level are good measures of successful resuscitation.

Either salt solutions or colloids can be used for bleeds of around 1000 ml. The main aim is to restore circulating volume. Larger bleeds require blood and other fluids to restore both volume and oxygen carriage.

Management of significant bleeding must always involve a surgeon.

Need for red cells depends on haemoglobin level, expectation of haemorrhage and general health. Frusemide is unnecessary with *at least* 90% of red cell transfusions.

The risk of catching AIDS from a unit of blood in Britain is about 1 in 10 000 000 – roughly the same as being struck by lightning. The other hazards of blood transfusion are more significant and you should know them.

Jehovah's Witnesses and their beliefs very rarely cause trouble, but when they do *get your consultant.*

The diagnosis of haemorrhage

Surprisingly, it can be difficult to recognize that a patient is bleeding. Even if the haemorrhage is external it is difficult to assess the amount lost (it is usually underestimated). When the blood is swallowed, or lost into the GI tract, joints or retroperitoneal space the loss may be occult.

Because of this difficulty, physical signs must be used to estimate the blood loss. However, single readings can be misleading. It is essential to record serial vital signs so that a trend or a response to therapy becomes apparent. Signs of haemorrhage are:

- **Blood pressure.** The systolic pressure tends to fall with haemorrhage, but healthy patients compensate so well that this only occurs after a substantial loss ($\geq$30% of blood volume). An earlier change is an elevation of the diastolic pressure due to vasoconstriction so that the pulse pressure (systolic minus diastolic) is narrowed. A low blood pressure should be recognized as a late sign of major blood loss.

- **Pulse.** The rate increases with blood loss, but again only after a serious loss ($\geq15\%$). Tachycardia of >120 b.p.m. represents a loss of $\geq30\%$. Bradycardia may supervene immediately before death.
- **Urine output.** This is an important indicator of perfusion of the kidneys and, by extrapolation, of other vital organs. An output of <0.5 ml/kg/h should cause worry and represents a loss of 30% if due to haemorrhage alone.
- **Level of consciousness.** Like urine output, this is a measure of perfusion of an organ system. A loss of 15% leads to anxiety (in the patient), 30% to confusion and 40% to lethargy or coma.
- **Respiratory rate.** For obscure reasons to do with physiological dead space, the rate increases.
- **Skin signs.** Pallor, slow capillary refill (normally <1 sec) and reduced skin turgor may all be useful pointers.
- **CVP/JVP.** These are difficult to assess and may even be misleading as venoconstriction in response to bleeding may elevate the CVP. Repeated measurements and careful charting are needed to make any sense of central pressures.
- **Haemoglobin.** The *concentration* of haemoglobin does not fall in acute haemorrhage because red cells and plasma are lost in their normal proportions, therefore a normal value does not exclude major blood loss. Only as *dilution* occurs (either physiologically or iatrogenically) in an attempt to restore the plasma volume does the haemoglobin concentration fall.

Changes in haemoglobin concentration can therefore only be used to assess bleeding in the long term and only if a separate assessment of *volume status* is made.

Establishing the cause

Surgical lesions
By far and away the commonest reason for bleeding is a hole in a blood vessel. Sometimes this can be diagnosed by inspection alone, but some sites (notoriously the pelvis and the retroperitoneum) can hold vast amounts of blood without external evidence. Diagnosis and treatment are often combined in exploratory surgery, so it is essential to involve a senior surgeon from the outset in all cases with unusual blood loss. Remember the possibility that drains may block; a dry drain does not exclude bleeding.

Bleeding tendency
A bleeding tendency or coagulopathy is rarely the prime cause of bleeding in surgical patients, but may co-exist or supervene as the situation deteriorates. Coagulopathy may have existed before surgery (and, with any luck, may have been detected, see Chapter I.10). Principal causes of coagulopathy after surgery are:
- *Dilution* of platelets or clotting factors by transfusion and fluid therapy
- *Inhibition* of platelets or clotting factors by drugs
- *Consumption* of platelets or clotting factors by DIC (disseminated intravascular coagulation) or cardiopulmonary bypass.

The diagnosis of a bleeding tendency is purely clinical; look for bleeding at venepuncture sites, expanding or fresh bruises, bleeding mucosa, haematuria and haemarthroses. Laboratory tests are used to help define the cause and to guide therapy.

- FBC: haemoglobin concentration is discussed above. Platelet count falls with dilution or consumption and is a useful early marker of DIC. A normal platelet count does not guarantee normal platelet function. A count of $<50 \times 10^9/l$ in the presence of a clinical coagulopathy definitely requires treatment. Changes in white cell count (up or down) are too non-specific to be of immediate use but trends may suggest an underlying cause (e.g. infection).
- PT: prothrombin time. Often expressed as INR (International Normalized Ratio), this is prolonged when factors VII, X, V, prothrombin or fibrinogen are deficient, or during warfarin therapy. Dilution, DIC or liver disease prolong the PT.
- (A)PTT: (activated) partial thromboplastin time is affected by deficiency of any factor except VII, and may be abnormal following dilution, DIC, heparin or warfarin therapy.
- LFTs: the liver is the major source of clotting factors and severe disease at a cellular level results in a mixed factor deficiency.
- FDPs: fibrin degradation products may be present in abnormally large amounts when haemostatic homeostasis has failed. This is found in acute consumption coagulopathy (DIC).
- U&Es: these are measured primarily as a baseline but also because urea is a platelet inhibitor.
- Ionized calcium: hypocalcaemia is a *rare* cause of coagulopathy following massive transfusion (see below). When testing for calcium, a tourniquet should not be used as it falsely elevates the result. Other sources of error are temperature, pH and protein concentration fluctuations. The best assay to request is the *ionized calcium* concentration, as this measures the physiologically active fraction of the total plasma calcium and is relatively free from error.

Principles of treatment

Whatever the cause, bleeding can be treated with a three-pronged attack: prevention of further haemorrhage; supportive treatment; and definitive treatment.

Preventing further haemorrhage

Elevation of the bleeding site is effective, particularly for venous bleeding. Whilst wearing gloves, apply direct pressure using any clean linen or swabs. Occasionally pressure on a feeding artery (e.g. femoral) may control a distal bleed. Tourniquets should not be used; they often increase venous congestion and bleeding and may threaten tissue viability below the constriction. Attempts to clip or tie bleeding points in a wound will disturb any clot and are unlikely to succeed except in the hands of experts and in the controlled conditions of the theatre.

Supportive treatment

The causes of death in bleeding are hypovolaemia and loss of oxygen-transporting capability. **Restoring plasma volume** is the first priority. Different types of fluid are differently distributed through the body (see Chapter II.6) and this determines the volumes needed.

- *Dextrose* solutions have no value in treating hypovolaemia because they are spread through the total body water.
- *Salt* solutions (saline, Ringer's, Hartmann's) are all useful, but only 30% of the volume stays in the circulation, the rest is distributed in the interstitial space.
- *Artificial colloid* solutions (Haemaccel, Gelofusine, Hespan, dextran) are confined to the circulating volume in the short term and thus less is needed to reverse hypovolaemia. Dextrans are best avoided in this situation as they have a platelet inhibitory action and can interfere with later cross-matching.
- *Blood products* (whole blood, packed cells, fresh frozen plasma, albumin, platelets) are also colloids and restore volume. Blood is a valuable resource and is indicated to restore both volume *and* oxygen carriage, but not to restore volume alone. When packed cells are used, extra fluid is given to make up for the extracted plasma (~200 ml/unit), in SAGM blood this volume has already been replaced in the transfusion lab. Similarly, FFP, platelets and albumin are not *primarily* indicated for restoring plasma volume.
- *Inotropes* are not used to treat hypovolaemia.

Restoring oxygen carriage is the second priority. Hypovolaemia causes hypoxia so all these patients need an oxygen mask. As bleeding continues and you successfully treat the hypovolaemia, *haemodilution* occurs. A rule of thumb is that a 500 ml blood loss leads to a 1 g/dl drop in haemoglobin concentration in a normal adult, *if treated with fluid replacement*. Untreated bleeding does not decrease the haemoglobin concentration, as discussed above. In the situation of acute bleeding it is desirable to preserve a haemoglobin concentration of around 10 g/dl. Therefore, if a 70 kg patient had a haemoglobin concentration of 12.5 g/dl before bleeding (for example) and lost 1000 ml of blood he would require fluid resuscitation, but probably not red cell transfusion.

Other blood products are often indicated:
- fresh frozen plasma to replace clotting factors;
- platelet transfusions for thrombocytopenia;
- other products like cryoprecipitate in certain circumstances.

Use of these expensive items is discussed below.

Monitoring progress is essential to diagnose continued bleeding and to avoid overtransfusion. Move the patient to a high observation area of the ward and start regular, frequent measurements of pulse, BP, respiratory rate (at least every 15 min) and urine output. You will need to catheterize the patient and ask for a burette-type collection bag. Repeated measurement of haemoglobin concentration will be needed to ensure adequate red cell replacement. Patients receiving high volumes of fluid, especially blood, are at very high risk of hypothermia and must be protected with blood-warmers and overhead heating or a hot air blanket (see Chapter II.20). At this time, it is worth reviewing the drug chart and discontinuing anything that worsens bleeding (non-steroidals, warfarin, heparin). When there is any suspicion of a coagulopathy discontinue all intramuscular injections.

Definitive treatment
All serious cases of postoperative bleeding will require you to call for help.

Usually this will be from a senior surgeon, as the definitive care is often exploratory surgery. In a few cases, surgery is needed as the only way of controlling haemorrhage and must be carried out even as resuscitation is continued. *Always get a surgeon involved early in any postoperative bleed.* More rarely, bleeding is due to a coagulopathy. Blood products may then be part of the treatment (see below). You are still likely to need advice from either a haematologist or from ITU.

Bleeding in children

The principles of diagnosis and treatment are the same as for the adult but there are important differences in interpretation of vital signs and in fluid volume calculations.

Physiological differences
Children normally have a faster pulse (150 in an infant to 100 at puberty). They have lower systolic blood pressures (80 for an infant to 100 at puberty). The respiratory rate is higher (from 40 to 20 with increasing age). The relatively large surface area of the child makes hypothermia more of a threat. The normal urine output is higher (1 ml/kg/h). The child is even better able than the adult to maintain a normal blood pressure despite serious hypovolaemia; hypotension must alert you to life-threatening bleeding. The early signs of shock in a child are poor skin perfusion and tachycardia.

Volume calculations
It is acceptable to assume that most adults are roughly the same size; children come in different sizes. The simplest measure of size is weight. Approximately 8% of the weight is blood. A blood loss of 200 ml is pretty serious to a 10 kg child (it's a quarter of the total blood volume), but not to an adult (blood donors routinely give 500 ml and can be resuscitated with tea and biscuits). Fluids given by the doctor must also be appropriate to the size of the patient. A suitable first fluid bolus to reverse shock is 20 ml/kg of salt solution. Monitor progress; if the apparent shock persists, repeat the bolus. Beware! You have now given 4% of the body weight, or 50% of the blood volume as crystalloid; this should make you suspect ongoing blood loss. If 30% of blood volume is lost (2.5% of body weight) it is likely that transfusion will be needed. Give blood in doses of 10 ml/kg with meticulous charting of signs.

Transfusion

Where does donated blood come from?
From volunteers aged 18–65, non-pregnant, in good health. Payment of donors, as in the US, encourages a higher risk donor population and concealment of aspects of medical history. Usually around 450 ml is taken at each sitting, and donors may give blood two or three times a year. Blood donations may not be accepted from healthy individuals with a history of recent foreign travel (malaria), those from high-risk groups (HIV) or those within 2 years of contracting glandular fever.

Once collected, blood is screened for hepatitis B antigen (HBsAg), hepatitis C antibodies (anti-HCV), anti-HIV antibodies and syphilis. Testing for cytomegalovirus (CMV) is also carried out, although CMV-positive blood can be safely given to all patients except in special circumstances, such as immunosuppression.

What happens to it?

Whole blood from a donor is collected into a bag containing citrate, phosphate and dextrose (CPD). Whole blood itself can be used for transfusion, especially in acute haemorrhage, but it is more practical to give the various components as they are required. Thus, the blood is fractionated into red cells and plasma.

Red cell transfusion

There are two basic indications for transfusion of red cells: acute haemorrhage and anaemia.

Acute haemorrhage: this is dealt with above.

Anaemia: where possible, anaemia should always be treated with the appropriate haematinics (iron, folate, vitamin B_{12}) before embarking on red cell transfusion. Most surgical patients with anaemia are iron-deficient. Often, however, transfusion is required because either the patient has not responded to haematinics, or rapid correction is required (e.g. to prepare for surgery).

The decision to transfuse depends on:

1. *The haemoglobin concentration.*
2. *The expectation of further blood loss.* This is one reason behind preoperative transfusion.
3. *The patient's general health.* Anaemia places greater demands on the heart, which must pump harder to maintain the same oxygen delivery. Patients with angina or myocardial dysfunction are less able to tolerate this, and a higher threshold for transfusion should be adopted for such patients.

A healthy patient who is unlikely to bleed can tolerate a haemoglobin of 8 g/dl without need for transfusion.

Patients with chronic renal failure are commonly anaemic for the lack of the renal hormone, erythropoietin. They should not be transfused before surgery unless actively bleeding. Transfusion carries additional hazards in this group, and has not been shown to be beneficial.

Blood should be warmed (at *least* to room temperature) and a unit can be given over 2–3 h in healthy patients. A venflon of 18 gauge (green) or bigger is required. Frusemide is only rarely indicated (see below). Regular 'blood obs' (temperature, BP, pulse, resps) are carried out during transfusion, so if you want your patient to sleep, don't transfuse overnight if you can help it. Blood giving sets contain a filter to remove aggregated red cells. Smaller additional filters are unnecessary. One unit of red cells will usually raise the haemoglobin concentration by 1 g/dl, though in frail elderly patients it may up it by 2–3 g/dl. Finally: if *you* hang a unit of blood, *you* check it.

Plasma products

The main plasma product used in the perioperative period is fresh frozen plasma or FFP. Each unit is the plasma derived from a unit of whole blood, which is rapidly frozen to a temperature of −30°C. The main indication for its use in the perioperative period is for the replacement of clotting factors. This is required in two common situations:

1. To correct the coagulopathy that accompanies massive transfusion;
2. To rapidly correct anticoagulation with warfarin.

Supplies of FFP are limited, and jealously guarded by haematologists, who use it to extract the products that they use to treat all the *interesting* haematological conditions. Consequently, documented coagulation defect is usually required before it is issued. The counter argument is that coagulation screens take time (1–2 h, usually), and anyway it is extremely rare for a patient to receive 6 units of packed cells and *not* have a coagulopathy. FFP takes a while to thaw out (20–40 min).

My advice is always ask for 2 units of FFP whenever you hurriedly cross-match 4 or more units of blood. They may or may not give it to you.

Platelets

The decision to transfuse depends on platelet count and whether or not the patient is bleeding. It is very rare for platelet transfusion to be required where the platelet count is $>50 \times 10^9/l$. If the patient is not bleeding, counts as low as $20 \times 10^9/l$ are acceptable. Always seek the advice of a haematologist before requesting platelet transfusions, especially if the cause of the thrombocytopoenia is not clear.

Platelets should not be given through filtered giving sets. Either use the simple filterless sets, or draw them up into a 50 ml syringe and inject by hand.

Preoperative cross-matching

Blood is usually cross-matched prior to routine surgery where significant blood loss is anticipated. For operations where transfusion is possible but unlikely, it is customary to send a sample for 'group and save' only. The sample is tested for atypical antibodies, and if none are present no blood is cross-matched unless it becomes necessary. Where atypical antibodies are found, appropriate 'antigen-negative' blood is obtained and reserved. Surgeons and anaesthetists should be made aware if there is an anticipated difficulty with cross-match, as it may be preferable to delay surgery.

Autotransfusion

The risks and expense of giving other people's blood has led to imaginative ways to use the patient's own red cells instead.

1. *Predeposit.* The patient donates blood at weekly intervals before surgery; this is stored in the normal way. This system requires considerable (dare I say unprecedented) co-operation between surgery, anaesthesia, blood transfusion service, haematology and hospital admissions. In addition, mismatch is still a risk (from clerical error) and it is contraindicated in those with sepsis, cardiac disease or anaemia. It is rarely used.
2. *Preoperative haemodilution.* The patient donates up to 2 units in the anaesthetic room, which is replaced by an equivalent volume of colloid. This yields two units of fresh, whole blood, containing useful levels of clotting factors and platelets. The hazards of transfusion are considerably reduced, but the risk of accidental mismatch remains.
3. *Blood salvage techniques.* Blood from the operating site can be collected into such 'cellsaver' devices, where it is anticoagulated, filtered and

washed, before being given back to the patient. Blood from wounds contaminated by pus or bowel contents cannot be used. The returned blood contains no plasma or platelets. The equipment is expensive, however, and the cost of salvaged blood is usually greater than bank blood.

Complications of blood transfusion

Fluid overload
Any i.v. infusion can precipitate fluid overload if you're not careful. The body responds to severe anaemia with varying degrees of high-output cardiac failure, and such patients may tolerate fluid loads poorly. Elderly patients, those with known cardiac disease, and those with megaloblastic anaemia are particularly at risk. The answer in this situation is to treat chronic anaemia with packed cells (you're unlikely to get whole blood anyway) and to give it slowly (e.g. 1 unit over 2–3 h).

Most recommend concomitant use of diuretics with transfusion, which can lower the risk of fluid overload, but this practice has been incorporated as a kind of brain stem reflex when prescribing blood. It is not necessary for every patient, and if you really must give a diuretic, frusemide 20 mg orally with every other unit of blood is plenty.

Infection
Transmission of infection by bacteria, parasites or viruses is a possible, but rare consequence of transfusion in the UK. The emergence of HIV has highlighted the risk, but infection prevention mechanisms have always been a part of the transfusion service. The key to prevention is the combination of rigid screening of donors and laboratory tests on donated blood. You will frequently be asked about the risks by patients.

Table II.7.1 shows the most important potential infections.

Immunological complications
ABO incompatibility. The ABO system consists of red cell antigens anti-A and anti-B. These antibodies are found in subjects who have never been exposed to the corresponding antigen and are thus called 'naturally occurring' antibodies. If, for example, the A antigen (e.g. blood from a patient with blood group A) is presented to a patient with anti-A antibodies (e.g. a patient with blood group O or B) the antibodies bind to the cell surface, and activate the complement cascade leading to a generalized haemolytic reaction, which may be fatal.

In a conscious patient, the transfusion of even a few millilitres of incompatible blood may cause dramatic symptoms: abdominal pain, vomiting, substernal pain and a feeling of restlessness and oppression. This may be accompanied by hypotension, haemorrhage, oliguria, multiorgan failure and death. In spite of strict procedures to avoid mismatch, such reactions occur with up to 0.2% of transfusions. The usual cause is failure to identify the patient correctly, either when labelling the sample or giving the blood, and is most common in times of stress (e.g. major trauma).
Rhesus incompatibility, and other red cell antibodies. Reactions may occur as a result of other red cell antibodies, the most important of which are rhesus anti-D reactions. These antibodies are so-called 'immune' antibodies and

Table II.7.1.   Key potential infections of blood transfusions

Viruses	HIV	Blood is routinely screened for anti-HIV antibodies, and the majority of cases of infection pre-dated this practice. There is still a risk if blood is taken from an infected donor before he/she has seroconverted, in the so-called 'window' period. The risk of infection at present is said to be ~1 in 10 000 000. The incidence in much greater in the US where the donor population is higher risk.
	Hepatitis B	The incidence of infection is ~1 in 100 000.
	'Non-A, non-B'	The identification of the hepatitis C virus, and the introduction of screening in 1991 has dramatically reduced the incidence of so-called 'transfusion hepatitis'. The incidence is ~1 in 100 000. There are probably other agents yet to be identified which can transmit hepatitis, but their relative importance is small.
Bacteria	*Staph*. etc.	Contamination is possible at the time of donation, but the storage procedure destroys most organisms. Transfusion of contaminated blood can, however, cause rapid septicaemia which may be fatal. Some organisms may have been present in the donor (e.g. *Salmonella, Yersinia*) and cause cross-infection. The incidence of bacterial infection after transfusion is ~1 in 1 000 000.
	T. pallidum	Syphilis may be transmitted in fresh blood (it is inactivated after 72 h of storage). Donor blood is thus screened for it. The importance has waned in the UK.
Parasites	Malaria	There are still occasionally cases of malaria infection by blood transfusion, and is a differential diagnosis of weird fevers occurring after blood transfusion.

occur as a result of prior exposure to the corresponding antigen. Incompatibility reactions do not lead to the activation of complement, and are mild, often merely causing a fever. Occasionally, such incompatibilities may cause a delayed haemolytic reaction, a week or so after transfusion. These reactions may cause anaemia and jaundice, but are not as severe as the immediate ABO reactions.

It is important not to expose a rhesus-negative woman of childbearing potential to rhesus-positive blood, to avoid the possibility of rhesus haemolytic disease of the newborn in the future.

Other reactions. Stored blood products contain a variety of foreign antigenic material which may cause mild reactions. White cells and plasma antigens are the commonest culprits. Fever is the commonest response, and mild episodes can be managed by slowing the transfusion and giving aspirin. Reactions to plasma proteins may cause urticaria, for which symptomatic treatment is indicated.

Other complications
- Coagulopathy, since stored blood contains very small quantities of coagulation factors.
- Hypothermia, if you are foolish enough to give blood at 4°C without warming it first.
- Citrate toxicity. Citrate is normally metabolized quickly, but may accumulate in massive transfusion in a very shocked patient, leading to hypocalcaemia and acidosis.
- Hyperkalaemia. Potassium leaks out of stored cells which lack the energy substrates to maintain the usual ionic gradients across the membrane. Normally, the potassium is rapidly reabsorbed, but in massive transfusion it may accumulate.
- Impaired oxygen delivery. Stored blood progressively loses 2,3-DPG and, without it, the oxyhaemoglobin dissociation curve is shifted to the left. In other words, although the haemoglobin carries oxygen beautifully, it does not offload it at the tissues. Blood stored for <14 days still has useful levels of 2,3-DPG.

Jehovah's Witnesses

Jehovah's Witnesses are a Christian sect whose religious beliefs occasionally conflict with the beliefs of doctors.

Although they accept all other forms of contemporary medicine, Jehovah's Witnesses do not accept autologous blood transfusion. The basis for this is their interpretation of certain passages of the Bible, and for any true believer it is not negotiable. Consequently, most are prepared to die rather than receive someone else's blood. Consent forms are available for the Witness to sign which absolve the doctor of responsibility for any adverse outcome attributable to withholding blood transfusion. In addition, many now carry legally enforceable advanced directives to prevent blood being given should they be unable to voice opposition at the time.

Legally and morally, your own opinions on the wishes of Jehovah's Witnesses are irrelevant. You have the right to refuse to treat a patient electively if you consider the risk of the procedure without blood outweighs the benefits. However, it is unacceptable to give blood products to a Witness without their express consent. Witnesses who have been given blood in this way describe it as being akin to rape, and it is a well-recognized cause of suicide among Witnesses.

There are some ways round the problem that are acceptable to Witnesses. Autotransfusion is acceptable, but only if a continuous circuit is maintained at all times. Hence, preoperative donation and haemodilution is OK provided the donated units remain connected to the patient's i.v. tubing at all times. Cellsaver, and pre-donation are usually not accepted. There is no religious objection to 'artificial haemoglobin', but the clinical effectiveness of these agents has been disappointing. Most hospitals now have Jehovah's Witness liaison committees, which can give more specific advice in such circumstances. Serious problems with the treatment of Witnesses are in fact extremely rare.

Most important of all, if a Witness is admitted with life-threatening haemorrhage, **senior** (i.e. consultant) assistance should be obtained **early**. This is especially necessary when the patient is a child, unconscious or when there is doubt as to the true wishes of the patient. Often family members or friends will press hard for the withholding of blood, but do not assume that the patient is a devout Witness without hard evidence.

Chapter II.8

FEEDING

Chapter II.8

FEEDING

KEY POINTS

Malnutrition is common in surgical patients, and leads to impaired wound healing, reduced respiratory function, increased susceptibility to infection and increased mortality. Any patient who is unable to eat normally for more than a few days should receive some form of artificial feeding.

Starvation in surgical patients results in breakdown of body proteins to provide substrate for gluconeogenesis. The stress of surgery or injury worsens the loss of nitrogen. Protein loss can be limited, but not prevented, in stressed patients.

Enteral nutrition is safe and effective, but requires the presence of a functioning gut.

Parenteral nutrition must be delivered through a central line and has many complications, particularly sepsis and hyperglycaemia. Parenteral nutrition must be monitored with frequent observations and laboratory investigations.

Dieticians can provide advice on any nutritional problem.

Introduction

Significant protein/calorie malnutrition is common in the hospital population, and is frequently unrecognized. Artificial feeding is a regular occurrence in surgical wards.

The reason to eat is to avoid the complications of malnutrition, which are of particular importance to the surgical patient:

- impaired wound healing;
- reduced resistance to infection;
- reduced respiratory function;
- anaemia;
- hypoproteinaemia and oedema;
- cardiomyopathy;
- longer convalescence and overall higher mortality.

Artificial feeding, either enteral or parenteral, should therefore be considered in any patient unable to eat for a couple of days or more.

The effects of starvation

The first response is to mobilize the stores of glycogen in the liver, which provides about 24 h worth of glucose. Although energy can be produced from other sources, glucose is always required to provide substrates for some organs, particularly the brain. Therefore, once the glycogen is used up, the body must make glucose via gluconeogenesis. The primary source of substrate for gluconeogenesis is amino acids, which are mobilized by the breakdown of body protein. Fat is also broken down to free fatty acids and glycerol. Fatty acids are metabolized via β-oxidation to produce useful quantities of energy, and ketone bodies which can also be used by the brain. With time, there are further hormonal changes that result in a drop in basal metabolic rate.

The nitrogen from protein catabolism is fed into the urea cycle, and eventually excreted in the urine, resulting in a negative nitrogen balance. In simple starvation it is relatively easy to reverse this catabolic state by providing nutrition.

The stress response

The situation of simple starvation refers to otherwise healthy individuals who just haven't eaten for a while. Most surgical patients, however, are subject to some degree of stress, in the form of surgery, injury, sepsis, etc.

The metabolic response to injury (the 'stress response') causes hormonal changes that differ greatly from the situation of simple starvation. The principal hormones released are:

Catecholamines	Cause increased protein
Glucocorticoids	catabolism, accelerated
Growth hormone	gluconeogenesis and
Glucagon	insulin resistance
Aldosterone	Cause salt and
ADH	water retention

There is, in addition, an *increase* in basal metabolic rate.

The extent of the stress response is related to the severity of the illness, and can be gauged by the degree of negative nitrogen balance. Whereas a non-stressed, starved patient may lose 5–10 g of nitrogen a day, in severe stress this figure may be as high as 30 g.

The stress response can be summarized thus:

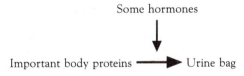

Unlike pure starvation, the negative nitrogen balance seen in stress cannot easily be reversed by providing nutrition, but with an appropriate feeding regimen the protein losses can be reduced.

The choice of regimen in stress is controversial. Some recommend tailoring nutrition to measured nitrogen loss, and giving energy in a fixed ratio (e.g. 80 kcal:1 g N_2). Most, however, prescribe the same for each patient.

Enteral nutrition

Tube feeding is indicated where there is a functioning gut and where swallowing is not possible. It can be administered via a normal nasogastric tube, but a fine bore feeding tube (e.g. Clinifeed®) is preferred for reasons of comfort. The position should be confirmed by X-ray before the tube is used. (Below the diaphragm is good, in the lung is bad.) Feeds can also be administered via a percutaneous gastrostomy tube ('P.E.G.'), which is preferred for long-term feeding, or a feeding jejunostomy. Tube feeding is safe, effective and helps to preserve gut function and integrity.

Occasionally a patient with a functioning gut (i.e. good bowel sounds and flatus) will not absorb nasogastric feed because the stomach won't empty. This problem can be circumvented either by the use of gastrointestinal prokinetic drugs (e.g. cisapride 10 mg tds p.o. or metoclopramide 10 mg tds p.o.), or by placing the feed straight into the jejunum. This can be done either by endoscopically placing a nasogastric tube beyond the pylorus, or with a feeding jejunostomy. Either way is better than unnecessary use of TPN.

The patient is fed with one of the many proprietary brands of solution, and each hospital has its own favourite. There is no need to bore you with the composition of each, but they all contain carbohydrate (usually as sucrose or glucose polymers), protein in the form of peptides or amino acids, triglycerides, electrolytes, vitamins, minerals and water. The nurses generally know what is normally used. If in doubt, pharmacists or dieticians can offer advice. The main complications of tube feeding are:

- Diarrhoea.
- Those of the tube insertion (malposition, oesophageal ulceration and perforation).
- Pulmonary aspiration, as it is commonly used in patients with impaired pharyngeal reflexes, and the presence of the tube promotes regurgitation.

It is traditional to begin with low strength 'starter' solutions, and then proceed to full strength. It should eventually be given by continuous infusion via an appropriate pump.

Diarrhoea can be managed by reducing the rate of infusion, switching to an iso-osmolar solution (most are anyway) or by treating symptomatically with codeine or loperamide.

Parenteral nutrition (TPN)

TPN is indicated when there is gut dysfunction, either due to ileus, fistulae or malabsorption syndromes. There are however, significant hazards with its use, and it is *contraindicated* where enteral feeding is possible.

TPN must be given through a central line, as its high osmolalilty will rapidly destroy any peripheral vein. Nothing else should be given in the same line because of the infection risk.

Choice of regimen

The junior surgeon should not normally have to prescribe complicated TPN regimens, except for the simple WDYNG[a] regimen. Usually, the regimen involves a bag of commercially prepared amino acid solution, a bag of dextrose and a bag of commercially prepared lipid solution. Vitamins and minerals are usually added.

[a] 'What do you normally give?'

500 ml of Synthamin 17® with 500 ml of 50% dextrose over 12 h
combined with 500 ml of 20% Intralipid® over 24 h.

In 24 h this gives:

Water (ml):	2500
Energy (kJ):	12 800
CHO (g):	500
Nitrogen (g):	14
Fat (g):	100

In many hospitals, the chosen feed constituents are added to a single bag
under aseptic conditions in the pharmacy. This makes administration more
convenient, and helps to prevent sepsis, and administration errors. Generally,
the prescription is written each day on a special order form.

Monitoring

To prevent metabolic complications, a system of monitoring for TPN
patients is essential. One suggested system is as follows:

- Regular observations: temperature, BP, pulse, respiratory rate, fluid
  balance.
- Regular ward testing: BM Stix, urinalysis.
- Daily: U&Es, glucose.
- Weekly (or more frequent): FBC, Coag screen, weight, LFTs, Ca, Mg,
  PO_4, C-reactive protein.
- As indicated: serum lipids, uric acid, blood gases, 24 h urine for urea and
  electrolytes.
- Special circumstances: N_2 balance, gas exchange, vitamin assays, trace
  element balance.

Complications

A list as long as an orang-utan's arm. A sample:

1. *Catheter complications*: pneumothorax, air embolus, thrombosis, vessel
   perforation.
2. *Sepsis*: TPN is an excellent culture medium. The line used for the feed
   should not be used for anything else, and should be changed regularly. If
   the patient develops a fever, the catheter should be removed and cultured.
   C-reactive protein is a sensitive marker of line infection.
3. *Fluid overload*: especially in the elderly or in cardiac or renal failure.
4. *Hyperglycaemia*: this is seen particularly in the stressed patient with
   insulin resistance (see above). Persistent hyperglycaemia should be treated
   with an insulin sliding scale or by reducing the infusion rate.
5. *Electrolyte imbalance.*
6. *Trace element deficiency*: especially in chronic therapy.
7. *CO_2 production*: i.v. glucose is converted eventually to CO_2. This can cause
   decompensation in patients with borderline respiratory function. Special
   preparations are available which provide a greater proportion of energy as
   lipid to avoid this problem.
8. *Spontaneous combustion*: not really.

Chapter II.9

BLOOD GASES

Chapter II.9

BLOOD GASES

KEY POINT

Don't panic.

Introduction

Confusion over the process of diagnosing an acid–base abnormality is rife. In this chapter, we will attempt to explain the subject by baring it down to the minimum relevant principles. This is not intended to be a comprehensive review, and purists will criticize the elementary approach taken here.

To reassure those of you with a delicate constitution, this chapter will **not** contain the words:

- 'Sigaard–Andersen'
- 'buffer–base pair' or
- 'because it just *does*, stupid'.

How to get a sample

Tools required are a 2- or 5-ml syringe, a 25-gauge needle, a steret and some heparin.

Draw up enough heparin to fill the dead space at the very end of the syringe (this is unnecessary with the special blood gas syringes). Choose a target vessel, preferably a radial artery, though brachial or femoral will do, and swab the skin. Feel the pulse proximal to the insertion point with your left hand. Using your right hand, insert the needle (with syringe attached) slightly distal to your fingers, at an angle of 45° pointing proximally. Stop advancing when you get a brisk flashback. The syringe may fill by itself, but you may need to draw back gently on the plunger. Arterial blood is usually bright red, but if your patient is bright blue, it won't be. Take about 2 ml then withdraw.

Finally, find an unsuspecting nurse, or a medical student you don't like, and get them to press on the artery for 5 min. They will inevitably have to listen to that 'Dracula' joke we are all so fond of.

Cap the syringe and label it. Always put the inspired O_2 concentration on the request form. If you are relying on your hospital's specimen delivery service, put the sample on ice. This will slow down the metabolism of cells in the sample, and reduce measurement errors. If you are taking the sample to the lab yourself, ice is unnecessary.

Acid–base physiology (abridged)

The activity of enzyme systems depends crucially upon the H^+ ion concentration, and thus maintenance of pH is essential for function of body tissues. H^+ is constantly produced by the body as a product of metabolism, and this extra acid must be disposed of without allowing pH to fluctuate. In order to minimize these fluctuations, the body uses **buffer systems**. Buffer systems reduce the free H^+ concentration...

$$\text{Strong acid + Buffer} \Longleftrightarrow \text{Weak acid + Salt}$$

...essentially by converting a strong acid into a weak one.

There are many buffer systems that operate within the body, but by far the most important is the bicarbonate system, which accounts for 60% of all ions buffered.

So:

$$H^+ + HCO_3 - \Longleftrightarrow H_2CO_3 \Longleftrightarrow H_2O + CO_2$$

...from metabolism   buffer   doesn't hang about long because...   it is rapidly converted to this

The reaction continues to move to the right, as long as CO_2 is removed

---

Important point no. 1: buffering is a temporary measure

The H^+ ions are still in the body. Further acid can only be mopped up by depleting bicarbonate, a finite resource. Removal of CO_2 only allows more buffering to take place. Definitive removal of acid from the body is only carried out by the kidney and the gut.

Conventionally, disturbances of acid–base balance are divided into two groups. Those in which the problem is to do with the production or excretion of acid, so-called **metabolic** disturbances, and those in which it is due to a problem with excretion of carbon dioxide, called **respiratory** disturbances.

Control mechanisms

You may remember the Henderson–Hasselbach equation:

$$pH = pK_a + \log [HCO_3^-]/[CO_2].$$

This basically shows that pH depends on the balance between bicarbonate and carbon dioxide.

Whenever a disturbance of acid–base balance occurs, the body will attempt to **compensate** for the abnormality, attempting to restore the pH towards normal. The normal respiratory system will respond to changes in pH with alterations in ventilation. The normal kidney will alter the excretion of acid depending on its availability.

Generally, the lungs can respond rapidly (i.e. within minutes) to changes in pH, whereas the kidney responds slowly (within days).

Important point no. 2 : the body never overcompensates for an acid–base disturbance.

Blood gas measurements

Blood gas results nearly always feature pH, P_aCO_2, standard bicarbonate, base excess and P_aO_2.

- **pH:** the most important. Tells you simply whether you have an acidosis or alkalosis. Normal range 7.36–7.44.
- **P_aCO_2:** tells you about alveolar ventilation, that is whether the patient is hyperventilating or hypoventilating.
- **Standard bicarbonate:** rather a confusing thing. Tells you what the bicarbonate would be if the P_aCO_2 were normal. Basically it is a measure of the size of metabolic disturbance.
- **Base excess:** this is more helpful. Base excess (or deficit) is a measure of the amount of acid (or base) required to restore the pH to 7.40, at a P_aCO_2 of 40 mmHg. Again it measures the magnitude of any metabolic component. Obviously, a negative base excess is the same as a base deficit.
- **P_aO_2:** the oxygen tension in arterial blood (see below).

Notice that standard bicarbonate and base excess, although derived differently, tell you basically the same thing.

Important point no. 3: ignore the standard bicarbonate

Interpretation

Blood gas measurement is really two tests in one: oxygenation and acid–base status.

Oxygenation
You don't have to be a rocket scientist to be able to interpret oxygenation, which is just a question of working out whether the P_aO_2 is low or not. There are one or two caveats, though.

1. Normal ranges. The 'normal' P_aO_2 for a patient breathing air is usually quoted as 80–100 mmHg (~13 kPa). P_aO_2 drops with age.
2. FiO_2. You cannot interpret oxygenation without knowing the inspired oxygen concentration. A P_aO_2 of 80 mmHg is OK on air, but if the patient is getting 80% oxygen, it certainly isn't. Note that unless the patient is breathing air, or receiving oxygen from a Ventimask, or a closed breathing system, it is impossible to know what the true inspired concentration is.
3. The oxygen saturation as given by the blood gas machine is a guess, based on the P_aO_2 and an assumed position of the oxyhaemoglobin dissociation curve. If the figure conflicts with that gained from a pulse oximeter, believe the pulse oximeter.

Acid–base status
The fundamental trick is to look at the pH and decide whether the changes in other values oppose the change in pH or not.

1. Look at the pH. Is it high or low?

    pH >7.44 = **alkalosis**
    pH <7.36 = **acidosis**

It is extraordinary how many intelligent people have difficulty with this concept.

2. Look at the P_aCO_2:

    P_aCO_2 >45 mmHg = hypoventilating
    P_aCO_2 <35 mmHg = hyperventilating

Now, try and fit them together. Given that high carbon dioxide makes you acidotic, decide whether the change in P_aCO_2 opposes or promotes the change in pH. If it opposes it, the disorder is metabolic. If it promotes it, the disorder is respiratory. So:

pH	P_aCO_2	Disorder
Low	High	Respiratory acidosis
Low	Low	Metabolic acidosis
High	High	Metabolic alkalosis
High	Low	Respiratory alkalosis

For goodness sake don't memorize this, *work it out.*
3. If you are still in any doubt, look at the base excess and fit that to the pH:

pH	Base excess	Disorder
Low	Large and negative	Respiratory acidosis
Low	Large and positive	Metabolic acidosis
High	Large and positive	Metabolic alkalosis
High	Large and negative	Respiratory alkalosis

Following this simple procedure, you will find that >99% of all blood gas results will clearly fit into the five basic categories: respiratory acidosis, respiratory alkalosis, metabolic acidosis, metabolic alkalosis or normal.

Arterial vs. venous sample
When arterial blood is difficult to obtain, and when the patient is sick, it is sometimes difficult to know whether you really took an arterial sample or not. There is no certain way to tell by looking at the result. The normal venous P_aO_2 is about 40 mmHg and the normal saturation 75%. Obviously, if your patient is very ill, the arterial values may be this low too. There are two pointers:
- If the P_aO_2 is much more than 50 mmHg (6.5 kPa), it is unlikely to be venous.
- If the measured oxygen saturation (from a pulse oximeter) is substantially greater than the guessed value on your blood gas result, it is unlikely to be arterial.

If doubt remains, you should repeat the sample.

Management of abnormalities

Metabolic acidosis
Typical blood gas result: pH 7.22
                                   P_aCO_2 21 mmHg
                                   Base excess −12
Causes:
1. Failure to excrete acid – renal failure.
2. Excessive production of acid – shock, post-cardiac arrest, ketoacidosis.
3. Excessive loss of bicarbonate – duodenal fistulae.
4. Weird stuff – acetazolamide therapy, renal tubular acidosis.
Management is directed at the cause.

Bicarbonate for metabolic acidosis?

Bicarbonate has been used almost without question for 50-odd years for any cause of metabolic acidosis.

$$H^+ + HCO_3^- \Leftrightarrow H_2CO_3 \Leftrightarrow H_2O + CO_2$$

too much of this

so add a bit of this. Great!

Increasingly, however, this practice has come into question. The commonest causes of acidosis, namely shock or cardiac arrest, are associated with poor perfusion and tissue hypoxia. Cells lacking oxygen are forced into anaerobic glycolysis with production of lactic acid. In this situation, giving bicarbonate is a bad idea:

$$H^+ + HCO_3^- \Leftrightarrow H_2CO_3 \Leftrightarrow H_2O + CO_2$$

Adding more of this is no good if...

...you can't get rid of this because of poor perfusion

Whereas bicarbonate can't get inside cells, carbon dioxide certainly can, where it makes the pH, and everything else, worse. Giving bicarbonate when there is tissue hypoxia impairs the uptake of oxygen, and worsens the acidosis.

Metabolic acidosis *without* tissue hypoxia is an indication for bicarbonate treatment. The two commonest examples are renal failure and acidosis from bicarbonate loss, as in bowel fistulae.

The amount of bicarbonate required can be calculated with the following formula:

Bicarbonate required (mmol) = base deficit × 0.3 × body wt (kg)

The 8.4% solution of bicarbonate contains 1 mmol/ml. It is sensible to give *half* the calculated requirement over about an hour first, then re-check the gases. Be aware that you are giving significant amounts of sodium. Bicarbonate should not be used for renal failure in the presence of fluid overload, as this is an indication for urgent dialysis.

Respiratory acidosis

It may be acute or chronic (or acute-on-chronic, where someone with bad lungs gets suddenly worse).

Typical blood gas result (acute):   pH 7.22
P_aCO_2 68 mmHg
Base excess 2

Typical blood gas result (chronic):   pH 7.32
P_aCO_2 68 mmHg
Base excess 12

The difference is that in chronic respiratory acidosis, the kidney has had time to compensate and the pH is nearer normal. The increased excretion of acid by the kidney leads to a large base excess.

Typical blood gas result (acute-on-chronic):   pH 7.22
P_aCO_2 75 mmHg
Base excess 12

Here, although the kidney has compensated for a degree of carbon dioxide retention, the P_aCO_2 is even higher than normal. The pH is low, therefore.

Acute respiratory acidosis is always serious, and senior assistance is urgently indicated as the patient may require artificial ventilation.

Common causes are:

1. Respiratory depression from drugs, such as opioids or sedatives.
2. Respiratory failure as a result of life-threatening asthma, pneumonia, etc.

Management of such problems is discussed in Chapter II.17

Chronic respiratory acidosis is less urgent. Patients with chronic lung disease, especially the 'blue bloater' type, may walk (or stagger) around with chronically elevated P_aCO_2. Urgent intervention is only indicated if there is rapid clinical deterioration. Patients with chronic respiratory acidosis may be subjected to 'hypoxic drive', and may drop dead if large amounts of oxygen are administered. See Chapter II.17 for details.

Metabolic alkalosis

Typical blood gas result: pH 7.55
P_aCO_2 43 mmHg
Base excess 14

Causes:

- Excessive bicarbonate administration: either i.v., or orally as in milk-alkali syndrome. This does not usually need specific treatment other than preventing further bicarbonate ingestion.
- Chronic potassium loss: lack of potassium in ECF means that the kidney relies more heavily on hydrogen ions to exchange for the sodium that has to be reabsorbed. To correct this may require many days' therapy, to replace the total body potassium levels (remember, most potassium is intracellular).
- Pyloric stenosis: where obstruction to the pylorus results in loss of acid without the loss of bicarbonate which normally accompanies vomiting.

The latter condition causes interesting biochemical disturbances. Initially, the body responds by reducing renal acid excretion, and bicarbonate appears in the urine. However, because of the persistent vomiting, sodium and water are also lost. In the presence of hypovolaemia, the kidney's need to reabsorb sodium overrides all other considerations.

Sodium can be reabsorbed in the following ways:

- Accompanied by chloride, however this is in short supply, being also lost in the vomit.
- In exchange for potassium. With a relative lack of acid around, this is the primary mechanism. Potassium depletion results.
- In exchange for acid. When potassium too becomes scarce, the kidney has no choice but to excrete acid in exchange for sodium. The urine becomes acidic, and the alkalosis gets worse.

The U&E results for such a patient will show raised urea and creatinine, reflecting dehydration, low potassium and low chloride, hence the term 'hypochloraemic alkalosis'.

True pyloric stenosis occurs only in neonates, but a similar clinical picture can occur in patients with severe duodenal ulceration. The definitive management is with a knife and fork, but the biochemistry can be tidied up fairly easily (and *must* be, before surgery):

- by giving sodium and water, to correct the dehydration;

- by giving chloride, to allow sodium to be reabsorbed without loss of potassium or acid;
- by giving potassium to correct the deficit.

This can be achieved with an appropriate volume of 0.9% saline with 40 mmol/l of potassium.

Specific treatment of the alkalosis itself is almost never required.

Respiratory alkalosis

Typical blood gas result: pH 7.55

P_aCO_2 21 mmHg

Base excess 1

There is only one cause: hyperventilation. This happens in:

- Lung diseases such as asthma, pneumonia, pulmonary fibrosis, mild pulmonary oedema. Treatment is directed against the cause.
- Hysterical overbreathing. In this situation, the lungs are normal. In many cases, the patient suffers the symptoms of hypocalcaemia, that is numbness and tingling in the fingers, even tetany and spasm. This is because alkalosis causes more calcium to bind to albumin, leading to a drop in *ionized* calcium. The symptoms are frightening, and exacerbate the hyperventilation. The treatment is to increase the P_aCO_2 by rebreathing. Get the patient to breathe in and out of a paper bag.

Chapter II.10

MONITORING DEVICES

Chapter II.10

MONITORING DEVICES

KEY POINTS

Non-invasive blood pressure measurement can vary between arms, and can be inaccurate if the cuff is not the right size. Automatic devices (e.g. 'Dinamap') underread at high pressures and overread at low pressures. They get totally confused when the pulse volume is variable as in atrial fibrillation, or when there is extraneous movement.

Arterial lines are very accurate. Don't inject anything down them or leave the cap open.

CVP lines need to be sited with the tip in the superior vena cava to give reliable readings. Confusion over interpretation of the results is widespread.

Pulse oximeters give information about oxygenation, heart rate and blood flow to the extremities. They should not be used to detect airway obstruction or hypoventilation, because the warning comes too late.

ECG monitors are best confined to medical wards or ITU, where the nurses are more likely to be able to recognize abnormalities. Patients at serious risk of dysrhythmias should be there anyway. The best 'first choice' monitors for a sick patient are a pulse oximeter and a Dinamap.

Introduction

Attitudes towards monitoring vary wildly. On the one hand, there is the very junior house officer, left to cope alone with an extremely sick patient, who rabidly monitors and measures absolutely everything, and believes the answers given by unreliable machines before trusting his own clinical findings. On the other, there is the old-school consultant who believes that all high-tech monitoring is the work of Satan, and clinical skills are all that are required.

The sensible approach is, of course, somewhere in between. With a small amount of basic knowledge of the function and limitations of the commonly used monitoring devices, they can become extremely effective adjuncts to patient care. However, monitoring should *never* be a substitute for clinical findings, and results should always be interpreted critically and fitted in with the **whole** picture.

Non-invasive blood pressure

Although non-invasive BP measurement is considered to be a fundamental clinical skill, relatively few clinicians are familiar with the factors that affect its accuracy. There is no 'gold standard' in blood pressure measurement, as all the available techniques are fraught with inaccuracies, and interpretation must take this into account.

The first problem with accuracy is that the pressure in different vessels varies as a result of the presence of vessel disease. The dimensions of the cuff in relation to the arm are important, and a narrow cuff on a fat arm will lead to an overestimate of blood pressure, and an excessively narrow cuff may lead to an underestimate. Auscultatory methods will be affected by the acuity of the clinician's hearing and, whatever you do, you are only intermittently measuring a very labile commodity.

Automatic blood pressure devices

These usually employ a technique called oscillometry. This works by inflating a cuff in the normal way, then measuring the tiny pulsations in the cuff as the pressure is reduced in a stepwise fashion. At each plateau of cuff pressure, the machine waits for two successive beats to ensure they are the same size. The onset of pulsations is taken as the systolic, the point at which they are greatest is the mean, and the point at which they disappear is the diastolic. The approximation to invasive arterial measurements is fairly good, although they tend to overread at low pressures and underread at high pressures. Fiddling with the cuff or moving the patient's arm will confuse it and give a dud reading (the movements caused by external cardiac massage often produce seemingly normal results).

It is important to realize, however, that they can be highly inaccurate where there is a wide variability of pulse volume, as in atrial fibrillation.

Arterial lines

These should only be used in a high-dependency unit. They are used for continuous pressure monitoring, and frequent blood sampling. Although there are sources of error, they are probably the most accurate means of blood pressure measurement when correctly set up. They also lead to surprisingly few long-term complications. The most important dangers are exsanguination (when someone leaves the cap open), and intra-arterial injection (when someone mistakes the line for an i.v.).

Central venous pressure monitoring

This thorny topic is dealt with in Chapter II.11.

Pulse oximeters

Few instruments have had as profound an effect on patient monitoring as the pulse oximeter. Introduced in the mid-1980s, they were quickly adopted for monitoring in anaesthesia, and have had a dramatic effect on safety. Since then, they seem to have spread to every corner of the hospital. They give reliable information about oxygenation, pulse rate and pulse volume, and can be small, portable and relatively cheap. As with any device, however, there are pitfalls.

Function
The basic principle of pulse oximetry uses the fact that haemoglobin and oxyhaemoglobin have different optical absorption spectra, that is they absorb light at various wavelengths differently. By passing light of two different wavelengths through a sample of blood and measuring the relative absorption of each, the proportion of oxygenated and deoxygenated blood, and thus the percentage oxygen saturation, can be calculated. The problem with *in vivo* measurement is that your finger contains a lot else besides arterial blood. Venous blood, muscle, connective tissue and bone, all absorb at least some of the emitted light. The pulse oximeter gets round this with sophisticated microprocessor data analysis, which manages to separate out only the pulsatile portion of the signal which is just the arterial blood.

Limitations
The pulse oximeter is extremely reliable but there are a number of instances when it may become misleading:
1. *Poor signal.* If the monitored digit is not well perfused for any reason, for example cold, arterial disease or shock, then the pulse oximeter may read nothing, or produce an inaccurate reading. Readings from cold hands can be improved by placing a rubber glove full of warm water under the patient's palm. Other sites may also work, the other hand, feet, or earlobe for example.
2. *Other forms of haemoglobin.* The pulse oximeter measures only the relative proportions of Hb and HbO_2, and assumes there are no other forms of haemoglobin present (carboxyhaemoglobin and methaemoglobin both have different optical absorption, um, thingies). This means that if there are significant amounts present, the pulse oximeter will give an inappropriately high reading.
3. *Dyes.* Large amounts of bilirubin or methylene blue in the blood will alter the reading. Some forms of nail varnish (Boots No. 7 is the worst culprit) may also affect the reading.
4. *Ambient light.* Strong light sources may confuse the photocell in the pulse oximeter probe.
5. *Venous pulsation.* This is important. You remember how the pulse oximeter cleverly picks out the pulsatile part of the signal, assuming it to be arterial. Patients in cardiac failure and others with tricuspid regurgitation, may have detectable venous pulsations which will reduce the average saturation reading. The typical venous saturation is about 75% so the effect is significant.

All is well....or is it?
Inappropriate usage may lead to a false sense of security:
- A pulse oximeter should **never** be used as a means of detecting airway obstruction as the warning will come far too late. This is a clinical diagnosis.
- A pulse oximeter will not necessarily detect hypoventilation if the patient is breathing oxygen. If the inspired oxygen concentration is high enough, people can be barely breathing with an O_2 saturation of 100%.

One final word. If there is a discrepancy between the saturation taken from the pulse oximeter, and that given on a blood gas result, believe the pulse oximeter – it is a *measurement*. The saturation from blood gases is a *guess* based on the measured P_aO_2 and an assumption of the position of the oxyhaemoglobin dissociation curve. The exception is a result from a lab which does co-oximetry on blood gas samples.

ECG monitoring

ECG monitors can detect dysrhythmias and ischaemia. However, before you decide to hook one up, ask yourself who will notice if abnormalities occur. Unless nurses are specially trained to recognize dysrhythmias, or unless you plan to camp out at the patient's bedside, an ECG monitor is just an expensive doorstop. For any unstable patient who you feel warrants closer monitoring, you are much better off with a pulse oximeter and a Dinamap. If the patient really is going to have serious dysrhythmias, they should be on CCU or ITU.

Chapter II.11

HYPOTENSION

Chapter II.11

HYPOTENSION

KEY POINTS

Definitions: no absolute figure can be given, systolic <90 mmHg is usually a cause for concern. Evidence of end-organ dysfunction (oliguria or confusion) is more important.

Causes: identifying the cause is essential to choosing treatment. The commonest causes are hypovolaemia, cardiogenic shock and sepsis, but there are many other causes that do not fit into these categories. Different aetiologies often co-exist, for example hypovolaemia and sepsis.

Assessment: begins with ABC: airway, breathing, circulation. If there appears to be time, detailed assessment of the notes, the patient and relevant investigations should be carried out. Fluid charts are useful, but be aware of the information that they **don't** give you.

CVP monitoring: useful if used correctly, dangerous otherwise. Do not get excited about individual measurements, but take seriously any changes, particularly in response to treatment.

Management: identify those **few** cases where a fluid challenge is not indicated and seek expert help. Give fluid to the rest. If things improve, repeat until haemodynamic variables and urine output are adequate. If things do not improve or get worse, seek help urgently.

Definitions

It is difficult to be precise about what exactly constitutes hypotension. The usual definition of shock from any cause requires some evidence of inadequate perfusion, as well as actual low blood pressure.

As the doctor on call, hypotension is whatever the nurse says it is until you have assessed the patient personally. Saying "Don't worry your pretty head about it" over the phone does nothing for your relationships with ward staff or your defence organization. Particularly if the nurse who calls you is a man.

As a rule of thumb though, the following should be cause for concern:

- systolic blood pressure <90 mmHg, or significant drop (e.g. 30 mmHg) from recorded baseline figure;
- ± evidence of end-organ dysfunction, for example low urine output, depressed consciousness.

Causes

The cause of a patient's hypotension is very important, as it can radically affect the management. Most textbooks trot out the usual stuff about four kinds of shock, as follows.

1. *Hypovolaemic shock.* Poor cardiac output is caused by inadequate pre-load.
2. *Cardiogenic shock.* Here there is a pump problem, due to poor myocardial contractility, dysrhythmia or mechanical disorders (as in valvular heart disease).
3. *Septic shock.* The condition of septic shock is a complex response to serious infection, that is a major cause of death on ICU. The root cause is probably the release of endotoxin from bacteria, although many other co-factors are involved. Initially, hypotension is the result of abnormal vasodilation with opening of arteriovenous fistulae, and there is a failure of tissues to extract oxygen. In this early phase, the patient usually has nice warm extremities, an otherwise unusual finding in shock. Later, there is overt myocardial depression. Septic shock is strongly associated with multiple organ failure and has a high mortality.
4. *Anaphylactic shock.* This is a specific situation caused by a type I hypersensitivity reaction and leading to massive release of vasoactive mediators such as histamine.

The problem with this approach, however, is that very few shocked patients fit neatly into a single category, and there are many causes of low blood pressure that do not fit into any. Restricting yourself to this rigid, exclusive, framework may hinder your attempts to rectify the situation.

Combined causes
The four principal aetiologies may co-exist with each other. For example, the patient with chronic heart failure, who is hypovolaemic after surgery. The failing heart is even more sensitive to lack of volume than the healthy heart, and may enjoy a bit of fluid resuscitation. In the early stages of 'sepsis syndrome' there is relative hypovolaemia, and fluid resuscitation is beneficial, whereas in advanced cases, there is direct myocardial depression, and the picture is closer to cardiogenic shock.

Other causes
There is a long list of causes of hypotension that do not fit into the above categories. Below is a sample.

- Drug actions: anaesthetic agents, analgesics, antihypertensive medication.
- Spinal/epidural anaesthesia: due to autonomic blockade.
- Vasovagal responses: patients can faint.
- Drug toxicity: for example digoxin, tricyclics or lithium.
- Pulmonary embolus: thrombus, air, fat or amniotic fluid.
- Measurement error: for example different pressure in each arm, excessively large cuff on a skinny arm.
- Pregnancy: for example caval compression in late pregnancy. Heavily pregnant women should not lie completely flat.
- Spinal shock: in a patient with recent high spinal cord injury.
- Hypothermia.
- Metabolic disorders: acidosis, disorders of calcium and phosphate, citrate toxicity.
- Addisonian crisis: for example a patient with undiagnosed Addison's, or someone who abruptly stops taking steroids.
- TUR syndrome: associated with hyponatraemia following transurethral resection. See Chapter II.22.

Assessment

Yes, I'm afraid you have to get out of bed. Assessment is aimed at deciding the cause and the severity of hypotension. Initial assessment, as always should begin with ABC:

- Airway – talk to the patient. If they speak to you the airway is clear.
- Breathing – check breath sounds, give oxygen, check respiratory rate.
- Circulation – is there a pulse? Rate and character? Insert a decent i.v. cannula (14- or 16-gauge). Is the hypotension severe or mild?
- Conscious level – awake and alert or comatose?

If you have ascertained that a cardiac arrest is not imminent, then you can revert to a more detailed assessment.

History

Age. Past medical history, both recent and long-standing. Surgical diagnosis if any, nature of any surgery, any reason for the patient to be actively bleeding? Fluid history. Look at the observation chart. Was the onset of hypotension sudden or gradual? Recently administered drugs, especially pain medications. Any specific symptoms, for example chest pain, breathlessness, itchy rash.

Examination

Look at the patient: pallor, cyanosis? Visible blood loss from drains or wounds? pulse, sweating, warm/cold extremities. Skin turgor. Measure the blood pressure yourself, manually, in both arms. JVP raised? Murmurs? Respiratory rate, Lung fields clear? Alert? Abdominal examination (including PR).

Investigations

Urine output (insert a catheter if necessary), FBC, U&E, cross-match (or at least group and save). ECG and/or chest X-ray if suspicions of cardiogenic component. CVP (see below).

The most familiar signs of shock (hypotension, tachycardia, pallor, oliguria, altered consciousness) provide a good estimate of severity, but are usually present whatever the aetiology and are not terribly useful when trying to assess the cause.

Central venous pressure monitoring

The measurement of CVP generates so much confusion and irrational behaviour that this little topic deserves a little section all to itself.

Measurement

CVP is measured using a catheter inserted into a central vein via subclavian, internal jugular or femoral approaches, or by threading a 'long line' up from an antecubital fossa vein. Note that a cannula in the external jugular vein will not give a reliable reading on account of the valve at its proximal end.

Although it is beyond the scope of this book to explain the techniques for CVP insertion, it is worth bearing in mind the potential complications of the procedure – haemorrhage and pneumothorax being the most common. Patients should always have a chest X-ray after CVP insertion to exclude air in the pleural cavity, and to ensure the catheter tip is where you want it (i.e. in the superior vena cava or right atrium). Catheters that thread up into the neck cannot be relied upon and should be re-sited. The other danger is air embolus: leaving the cap open risks drawing air into the circulation with potentially fatal consequences.

The catheter can then either be connected to an electronic pressure transducer, or more commonly to a fluid manometer line. Measurements of CVP should be taken at the end of expiration. When using a fluid manometer, take care not to fill up the vertical tube too far, as wetting the sponge filter in the top may affect accuracy. The reference point is the anterior axillary line in the 4th interspace (not the angle of Louis) – use a spirit level. The meniscus should fall and rise with respiration. To take a measurement, fluid is run into the vertical arm from a bag of crystalloid solution until the level is about 20 cm above the zero point. The three-way tap is then closed to the bag, allowing the fluid in the vertical arm to drain into the patient until equilibrium is reached. The height from the zero point gives CVP in cmH_2O.

Physiology

So what are we actually measuring?

CVP is used as a means of estimating ventricular filling and volume status. There is a long chain of assumptions between these concepts, however. Following this chain will help you to interpret CVP and avoid some of the commonest errors.

The chain starts with Starling:

The energy of contraction is a function of initial fibre length. This was determined from experiments on isolated heart muscle preparations. The more you stretch the muscle fibre, the harder it contracts.

Ventricular end-diastolic volume (VEDV) varies with stroke volume. This is the extension of Starling's principle to the heart as a whole, that is the more filled the ventricle, the better the cardiac output. This is broadly true, but the relationship for a healthy heart is different from that of a failing heart (see Figure II.11.1).

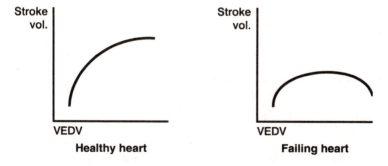

Figure II.11.1. Representation of Starling's principle in the healthy and failing heart.

In a healthy heart, more volume leads to more output. In the failing heart, however, the curve is bell-shaped, and higher end-diastolic volumes lead to *reduced* output. In this case, offloading the ventricle improves haemodynamic status.

VEDV *varies with volume status*. This is true up to a point. However, in low volume states, particularly in the young and fit, compensatory veno-constriction can maintain VEDV.

Ventricular end-diastolic pressure (VEDP) *varies with VEDV*. This is roughly true for any individual patient. Obviously, it is very much easier to measure end-diastolic pressure than end-diastolic volume. (When all you have is a hammer, everything starts to look like a nail.) VEDP is also known as 'filling pressure'.

Right VEDP *varies with left VEDP*. This is true in health, but you are unlikely to be measuring CVP in a completely healthy patient. A variety of disease states lead to a difference in function between the two sides of the heart. The most important are respiratory disease, mitral stenosis, cardiac failure and pregnancy. A higher than 'normal' CVP is to be expected in a patient with respiratory disease and does not necessarily signify fluid overload.

CVP *is the same as right VEDP*. To all intents and purposes, this is true.
You can see, therefore what an indirect measure CVP is.

Interpretation. To try and make sense of the previous section

1. The 'normal' CVP is about 5 cmH$_2$O in health, but healthy patients do not need their CVPs measured.
2. CVP is a very roundabout way of guessing left ventricular filling. There are many assumptions along the way so **absolute values are completely meaningless**. Do **not** base fluid management decisions on a single CVP reading.
3. CVP is often maintained in the 'normal range' over a wide range of volume states. Normal CVP does not rule out hypovolaemia or fluid overload.
4. For patients with heart failure, there is a level of CVP at which they are haemodynamically happiest. Your job is to find it. This 'optimum' CVP is very unlikely to be within the 'normal range'.
5. CVP is extremely useful when monitoring trends (e.g. steadily dropping CVP suggesting progressive hypovolaemia) or response to treatment.

Management

Once basic resuscitative measures have been taken (airway, oxygen, big drip) the cornerstone of the treatment of hypotension is the **fluid challenge**, and the key task of the assessment is to identify those (few) cases in which it is *not* indicated. The principle of the fluid challenge is an example of a servo loop, and its function is as much diagnostic as therapeutic.

Essentially, the procedure is to infuse 100–200 ml of fluid rapidly, and monitor the effects on heart rate, blood pressure, urine output and CVP. It doesn't greatly matter whether the fluid is crystalloid (e.g. 0.9% sodium chloride) or colloid (e.g. Gelofusine®, Hespan®, blood). A more rapid response might be expected from the colloid solutions which preferentially expand the intravascular compartment, but they are more expensive. Solutions of 5% dextrose or dextrose–saline are not particularly useful, as their effect on ECF and intravascular volume is much less.

If fluid therapy is indicated, then a favourable effect on haemodynamic variables will be seen, and further challenges should be given until the patient is adequately resuscitated. If there is a deterioration, then hypovolaemia is unlikely to be present.

There are, in addition, one or two caveats for the diagnosis and treatment of shock:

- Never, **never** diagnose 'fluid overload' purely on the basis of a fluid balance chart. Many important losses never get charted (e.g. fluid in small bowel, large expanding haematoma around a ruptured aorta, pre-existing deficit, insensible loss).
- Do not base your decisions on a single CVP reading.
- The management of haemorrhage is surgical, for which you need a surgeon.
- Blood should *always* be warmed when given rapidly. Cold blood is worse than no blood.
- Opioids are only rarely the sole cause of hypotension. However, when a hypovolaemic patient is given morphine for pain, the blood pressure may drop dramatically. The treatment is fluid, not naloxone.

When the fluid challenge works

If a fluid challenge produces significant improvements in any of the usual cardiovascular indicators, that is pulse, BP, urine output, CVP, then the process should be repeated as often as necessary to rectify the situation. However, at *each stage*, the patient should be re-assessed. Fluid overload, particularly in the elderly, is a hazard if fluid is given without regular assessment.

When the fluid challenge doesn't work

This occurs in three situations:

1. When the patient has true cardiogenic shock, with inadequate perfusion despite very high filling pressures. The management of this condition is likely to involve invasive monitoring, inotrope therapy, treatment of dysryhthmias and even cardiac surgery. It is therefore not something that a lone house officer should be tackling. You should contact your next on call and the ITU registrar for assistance.
2. When the cause requires a different form of intervention, for example in tension pneumothorax, cardiac tamponade or Addisonian crisis.
3. When hypovolaemia is so desperate that a small fluid challenge is inadequate to make a noticeable difference. Again, you need help here.

Chapter II.12

DYSRHYTHMIAS

DYSRHYTHMIAS

KEY POINTS

Immediate action: when faced with a possible dysrhythmia, check airway, breathing, pulse, give oxygen, ensure venous access, alert other staff. Measure blood pressure manually. Arrange a 12-lead ECG, find an ECG monitor. Look for underlying causes, send blood for U&E, gases and full blood count.

Diagnosis requires an ECG strip. Decide whether it is fast or slow, broad or narrow, regular or irregular.

Atrial ectopics are insignificant unless very frequent.

Ventricular ectopics usually don't require therapy but may herald worse. Worry if they are frequent, multifocal, occurring in runs or on the T wave of preceding beats. Lignocaine 100 mg i.v. is the first-line treatment.

Atrial fibrillation is very common. Most cases are chronic, normally well-controlled AF. Aim for a ventricular rate of 80 or below. Treat the obvious (e.g. pain) first. Definitive management is with digoxin, although in an emergency cardioversion can be considered. Check potassium before giving digoxin.

SVT is over-diagnosed. True SVTs occur often in young people with a history of palpitations. Physiological manoeuvres may help. Before using drugs, ensure that your 'SVT' is not in fact atrial fibrillation.

Atrial flutter is also common, and the management is similar to that for atrial fibrillation.

Ventricular tachycardia. Any broad complex tachycardia is VT until proven otherwise. The differential is tachycardia in someone with bundle branch block. If there is time, a 12-lead assists diagnosis. Treatment for VT with a pulse is lignocaine; without a pulse the treatment is defibrillation.

Sinus bradycardia may be normal, but can be treated with atropine fairly safely if not. Heart block of 2nd or 3rd degree is an indication for cardiological assistance.

Pacemakers, especially the older type, very occasionally malfunction under anaesthesia.

Introduction

Dysrhythmia is the correct term for abnormalities of cardiac rhythm. The term 'arrhythmia' refers only to that specific instance when the ECG monitor shows a straight line.

Dysrhythmias in the surgical patient are not uncommon. They are most often the result of pre-existing cardiac disease, but may occur as a result of other factors such as hypoxia, hypercapnia, hypovolaemia, drug actions, electrolyte or acid–base disturbance, or a combination of these. When faced with a patient who has or may have a dysrhythmia, your duty is as follows:

1. Make sure of all the ABC-type stuff: airway, oxygen, breathing, pulse, BP, conscious level, and decide whether hitting the panic button is warranted. Make sure the 'crash trolley' is nearby, and nursing staff are aware of the problem. Hypotension in the presence of dysrhythmia is an indication for urgent, expert help.
2. Get a 12-lead ECG, fish out the preoperative one for comparison, try to come to a diagnosis.
3. Exclude any underlying cause: give oxygen, establish i.v. access, send urea and electrolytes and blood gases.
4. Treat the dysrhythmia with specific therapy, or get someone to do it for you.

Diagnosis

Although clinical examination is mandatory, it is not much use in diagnosing the specific dysrhythmia. For this you need a rhythm strip, or better still a 12-lead ECG.

In reading an ECG strip, there are three simple things to decide:

1. Is it a tachycardia or a bradycardia?
2. Is it broad-complex (QRS >0.12 sec or three small squares) or narrow-complex?
3. Is it irregular or regular?

Figure II.12.1 provides an algorithm to help you diagnose the various different abnormalities.

Atrial ectopic beats

These are extra beats on a background of sinus rhythm, in which the QRS complexes are the same as normal beats, and the P waves (if visible) are different. They can occur in normal individuals, or be precipitated by caffeine, alcohol or stress (and are therefore more common in the junior doctor). Occasionally there is a more sinister underlying cause, such as electrolyte abnormality or drug toxicity (e.g. digoxin). Treatment is not usually necessary.

Ventricular ectopic beats

These are extra beats on a background of sinus rhythm, where the QRS complexes are different from normal beats. The QRS complexes are wide and bizarre, and not preceded by a P wave. They may be unifocal, where the abnormal QRS is always the same, or multifocal, where they are different.

Like atrial ectopics, they may be of no consequence, but should always be taken seriously if they are:

- frequent (i.e. >5/min);
- multifocal;
- occurring in runs of two or more;

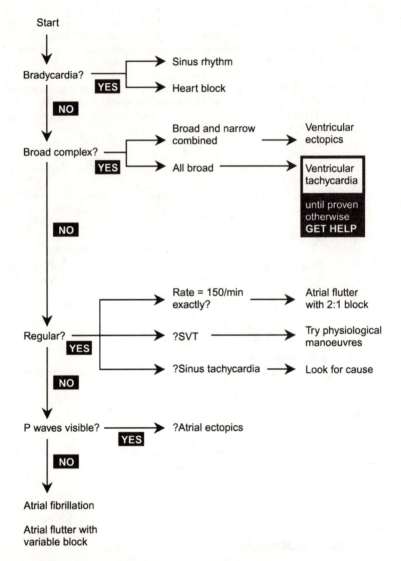

Figure II.12.1 Algorithm for the diagnosis of dysrhythmias.

- occurring at or just before the T wave, the so-called R-on-T phenomenon, which can precipitate ventricular fibrillation.

If so, an underlying cause such as electrolyte disturbance, ischaemia or hypoxia should be sought. Specific treatment is often indicated to prevent progression to more serious dysrhythmias. Lignocaine 100 mg (10 ml of 1%) i.v. is the first choice drug.

Atrial fibrillation

This is an irregular, usually narrow-complex tachycardia with absent P waves. It is the commonest dysrhythmia of the lot.

Long-standing AF is common in surgical patients, though acute onset AF can occur in myocardial infarction, thyrotoxicosis, pulmonary embolism, electrolyte disturbances and hypoxia. The commonest presentation of 'fast' AF postoperatively is in the previously well-controlled patient whose ventricular rate increases (to >100 b.p.m.). This may be a result of a lapse in the patient's regular digoxin dose (see Chapter I.3), or of the sort of problem that would send anyone's heart rate up, for example pain, hypovolaemia, etc.

Treatment is as follows:

- Treat pain, hypovolaemia, hypoxia.
- Check potassium before starting digoxin.
- For a undigitalized patient, a full loading dose of digoxin can be given i.v., but is often not necessary. Call medics for advice.
- For a digitalized patient, the usual problem is inadequate levels of digoxin, and a single extra dose (e.g. 500 mcg orally) will do the trick. **Digoxin toxicity** is possible, particularly in the presence of hypokalaemia. In this instance, however, the ventricular rate is usually low and ventricular ectopics are also seen.
- For a shocked patient use DC cardioversion.

Digoxin has a narrow therapeutic window, but undertreatment is more common than toxicity. Almost nobody on 0.0625 mg or 0.125 mg per day has levels in the therapeutic range. The important exception, however, is the patient with **renal impairment**, who requires a lower maintenance dose, though the loading dose is unchanged.

Paroxysmal atrial fibrillation

Some patients flip in and out of AF; so-called paroxysmal atrial fibrillation. Digoxin will not prevent paroxysms of AF, but will reduce the ventricular rate when they occur. The drug of choice is sotalol 120–240 mg/day, though the decision to treat should be deferred to a cardiologist.

Superventricular tachycardia (SVT)

SVT is a dumb name for this condition, and causes confusion because, technically, *any* tachycardia except VT is an SVT. What people normally mean by SVT is paroxysmal re-entrant tachycardia. On an ECG it is a regular, narrow-complex tachycardia, rate usually between 140 and 250 b.p.m. There are abnormal P waves with a fixed relationship to the QRS complex. It can be very difficult to distinguish SVT from sinus tachycardia, or from atrial flutter with 2:1 block. It is not particularly common in the postoperative period, but may be seen in otherwise healthy young patients, who may have a history of palpitations. It is the usual dysrhythmia seen in Wolff–Parkinson–White syndrome, and may occur after myocardial infarction.

A true SVT may respond to physiological manoeuvres, which are intended to terminate the dysrhythmia by provoking vagal activity. Carotid sinus massage is the best known technique, but the most effective is a sustained valsalva manoeuvre. The patient can be asked to blow into the manometer part of a sphygmomanometer, and asked to maintain a pressure of 20–30 mmHg for 10 sec and then breathe out. On exhalation, there is a burst of vagal activity that slows conduction in the AV node, and may terminate the dysrhythmia.

If drug treatment is required, the agent of choice is adenosine 3 mg i.v., followed by 6 mg then 9 mg if necessary. This drug inhibits AV conduction, and has the advantage of being very short acting. Adenosine is a powerful vasodilator, and transient hypotension is common with its use. Note that the commonest mistake is to use adenosine when the rhythm is really AF, which results in profound hypotension.

Atrial flutter

Flutter waves occur instead of P waves, usually at a rate near to 300/min, and give a sawtooth appearance to the baseline. There is usually a degree of block, that is not every flutter wave is conducted to initiate a ventricular contraction. Normally there is 2:1 or 3:1 block, or a mixture which gives an irregular pulse. A narrow-complex tachycardia at a rate very close to 150 b.p.m. is highly suggestive of flutter with 2:1 block. The management is as for atrial fibrillation, and is primarily aimed at controlling the ventricular rate, although amiodarone or DC cardioversion may restore sinus rhythm.

Ventricular tachycardia (VT)

VT is a medical emergency.

The haemodynamic effects of VT are variable. It can cause relatively little disturbance or lead to cardiac arrest and, if a firm diagnosis is made, senior help should always be sought.

Any broad-complex tachycardia is VT until proven otherwise. The main diagnostic difficulty occurs with other forms of tachycardia in patients who normally have bundle branch block, and whose QRS complexes are always wide. If this is suspected, the diagnosis can be confirmed by taking a 12-lead ECG and comparing it with previous traces. If the morphology in corresponding leads is similar, then VT is unlikely. VT is usually slightly irregular. The diagnosis can be confirmed if independent atrial activity can be spotted, that is regular P waves superimposed on the ventricular activity.

VT in a conscious patient is treated with lignocaine 100 mg (10 ml of 1%) i.v. in the first instance, followed by an infusion of 1–4 mg per hour. For patients who arrest in VT, the treatment is as for VF.

Bradycardias and heart block

Sinus bradycardia may be a normal finding in fit young individuals or during sleep. It is usually seen in patients treated with β-blockers. It may, however, be an ominous sign, particularly of hypoxia. If there is haemodynamic compromise in the presence of sinus bradycardia, and no underlying cause is immediately evident, it should be treated with oxygen and atropine, 0.3–0.6 mg i.v.

Occasionally, a bradycardia may be the result of heart block, where there is a problem with conduction of the impulse between atria and ventricles. It is a sign of significant underlying heart disease.

Heart block has three grades:

1. First degree, in which the impulse is delayed, but gets through each time. The finding on ECG is a long P–R interval (>0.2 sec). This is a sign of cardiac disease, but is not an urgent problem.
2. Second degree, in which atrial impulses are sometimes transmitted but not always. The most obvious abnormality is more P waves than QRS complexes. There are two subtypes: type I in which the P–R interval gets progressively longer until a beat is dropped (the Wenckebach phenomenon), and the more serious type II, in which the ratio of Ps to QRSs is more fixed (e.g. occurring in 2:1 or 3:1 pattern). Second degree heart block deserves urgent attention from a physician.
3. Third degree, in which none of the atrial impulses are conducted. On ECG, the P waves are regular, but bear no relationship to the QRS complexes. The ventricular rate is usually low. Third degree heart block occurs after myocardial infarction, or may be the result of degenerative changes in the conducting system. It can also be congenital. The definitive treatment is transvenous pacing but, as a temporary measure, the ventricular rate can be improved with an infusion of isoprenaline.

Chapter II.13

HYPERTENSION

HYPERTENSION

KEY POINTS

Definition depends on age. 'Normal' systolic is about 100 + age in years. Diastolic over 110 mmHg is too high. Any dramatic increase over baseline is important.

Sustained hypertension causes strokes and myocardial ischaemia.

Causes. Underlying causes **must** be treated before giving antihypertensives.

Treatment. Specific management in the postoperative setting has short-term aims. Let an expert decide whether to treat long term and what to use. Sublingual nifedipine is safe and effective. Intravenous labetalol is also useful, but must be used with caution.

Introduction

Hypertension is a common reason for being summoned in the perioperative period. Sustained severe hypertension is associated with serious complications such as myocardial ischaemia and cerebrovascular events. There is often an underlying cause which has to be identified and treated before any antihypertensive medication is given.

Definitions

As with the definition of hypotension, it is difficult to give absolute figures, and the definition will vary from patient to patient. Systolic pressure tends to rise with age, and a rule of thumb is that 'normal' is 100 + (age in years) mmHg. From this you can see that a systolic of 160 mmHg may be normal in an elderly patient, but abnormal in a 20-year-old. For diastolic hypertension, a figure of 110 mmHg is definitely abnormal, but in younger patients, it shouldn't really rise above 100 mmHg.

The other issue is that hypertension needs to be sustained to warrant specific therapy, that is more than one reading separated by a suitable length of time.

Causes

It is crucial to identify any underlying cause before instituting treatment. The following is a list of important causes, in rough order of importance:

- Pain: a very obvious and very common cause of hypertension. NEVER give antihypertensives to a patient in pain.

- Anxiety: so-called 'white coat hypertension'. Try reassurance before reaching for the tranquillizers.
- Drugs: dopamine and other inotropes, salbutamol, aminophylline infusions.
- Hypercapnoea/hypoxia: raised CO_2 causes direct vasomotor stimulation. Hypoxia causes agitation in the early stages, but later causes myocardial depression.
- Full bladder: especially in confused elderly people.
- Raised intracranial pressure: via the Cushing reflex.
- Malignant hyperpyrexia: pretty spectacular when it happens, but rare as rocking-horse do-dos.
- Hormonal: phaeochromocytoma, thyroid crisis, carcinoid. All rare.

Once the above have been excluded, the most likely cause is ordinary 'essential' hypertension. Normally, a well-controlled hypertensive should behave perfectly well during and after surgery, but blood pressure can get out of hand in the following circumstances:

1. Undiagnosed hypertension. Surgery is not an uncommon way for hypertension to present.
2. Hypertension that was inadequately controlled before surgery.
3. When the patient was mistakenly advised not to take their regular medication on the morning of surgery.

Treatment

Give oxygen. Assuming treatable causes have been treated, and hypertension appears to be persistent, it is time to consider drug treatment. It is not really necessary for the surgical house officer to choose a long-term anti-hypertensive regimen, as this can be achieved in the cold light of day by a physician, or the patient's GP. The goal is short-term control. After this, the problem may settle down, in which case no further intervention is necessary, or will recur, thus indicating the need for referral.

There are two drugs you need to know for this situation:

1. *Sublingual nifedipine.* This is quick, safe, easy to administer, can be given by nurses, has a useful duration of action and has very few contra-indications. The dose is 10 mg. Notice you need the *capsules* not the tablets. The patient should bite the capsule and keep the contents under the tongue. It should not be swallowed. It can even be written PRN on the chart (e.g. '10 mg S/L up to 2-hourly for systolic >170 mmHg'), thus promoting (your) REM sleep.
2. *Intravenous labetalol.* This should be considered for those who cannot take sublingual medication because of sedation, poor cognitive function or unco-operativeness (in which case consider pain or full bladder) or for those in which nifedipine is ineffective. Labetalol has both α- and β-blocking activity. Although β-effects predominate in chronic therapy, it is likely that the α-effect is most important in i.v. bolus administration. The dose i.v. should be titrated against effect, giving 5 mg to start with. If no effect is seen after 5–10 min, 10 mg can be given, then 15 mg, and so on. Remember that it is a β-blocker, and as such it is contraindicated in (all together now) *asthma and cardiac failure.*

Chapter II.14

MYOCARDIAL ISCHAEMIA

MYOCARDIAL ISCHAEMIA

KEY POINTS

Coronary artery disease is commoner than you think. It is the biggest killer of surgical patients.

Postoperative ischaemia may be 'silent', or may present in an atypical manner.

Mortality has been shown to improve if meticulous care is taken throughout the perioperative period. This boils down to closer monitoring, oxygen, analgesia and adequate fluid replacement.

Background

Ischaemic heart disease is common in the surgical population, and myocardial ischaemia is the single biggest killer in the perioperative period.

There is no doubt that postoperative myocardial ischaemia occurs more frequently than is recognized, and often it does not generate the typical signs and symptoms. Chest pain may be masked by analgesic or anaesthetic medication, or confused with incisional pain and, in many cases, ischaemia may be truly silent.

There is a constant risk that patients with reversible ischaemia may progress to infarction. Postoperative MI occurs most frequently 48–72 h after surgery and carries a poor prognosis. Much effort is usually taken to prevent ischaemic events in the heavily monitored environment of theatre, but such care rarely persists into the postoperative period.

However, it has been shown that careful handling of patients with ischaemic heart disease *throughout the entire perioperative period* can substantially reduce mortality. An approach, similar to that aimed at preventing DVT, should be adopted: identify those at risk, and employ a full range of simple measures to prevent ischaemic complications.

Patients at risk

Any of the following carry a high incidence of ischaemic heart disease, and are thus at risk:
- Previous MI, especially within 6 months, or known angina.
- Hypertensives, especially those with ECG evidence of left ventricular hypertrophy.
- Diabetics.
- The elderly.
- Vascular surgery patients.
- Smokers.
- Those with ECG evidence of 'strain', bundle branch block or old MI.

Prevention

There is nothing new or clever here. The priority is to avoid anything which upsets the balance of myocardial oxygen supply and demand (i.e. avoid tachycardia, hypotension, hypertension and hypoxia). Attention to detail saves lives.

1. *Fluid balance.* Ensure good hydration and adequate urine output. CVP monitoring is justified in complex situations. Avoid anaemia (haemoglobin level <10 g/dl).
2. *Analgesia.* Pain is very bad for the heart (see Chapters II.1–II.4).
3. *Oxygen.* Remember that patients are prone to severe hypoxia for 3 or 4 days after surgery, **particularly at night**. *Prescribe* oxygen for at-risk patients. Use nasal cannulae if the patient won't keep a mask on.
4. *Hypothermia.* Look for it, prevent it and treat it (see Chapter II.20).
5. *Regular medication.* Continue all antihypertensives and antianginal medication throughout the perioperative period. If the patient is not taking oral medication and you are having trouble providing parenteral therapy, ask a physician. Don't forget that GTN can be given as a transdermal patch.
6. *Monitoring.* The more the better, though this is obviously constrained by resources, nursing manpower and level of training. The usual observations (pulse, BP, temp, resps, urine output) definitely. Pulse oximeter or automatic BP if available.
7. *DVT prophylaxis.* Minihep and stockings, more important than ever (see Chapter II.23).

Management

For patients who present with the usual clinical picture of angina or MI (i.e. central chest pain, radiating to neck or arms, nausea, sweating, breathlessness), the management is as follows:

1. Examine for evidence of hypotension, failure or dysrhythmia.
2. Treat ischaemic chest pain with increments of i.v. morphine.
3. Employ measures 1–7 above.
4. Get a 12-lead ECG and compare with the preoperative trace. (Now you know why we always do a preoperative ECG.)
5. Send blood for cardiac enzymes. Creatine kinase (CK) levels are elevated after surgery, so you will have to ask specifically for the cardiac isoenzyme CK-MB.
6. Refer the patient to the physicians for further management. If MI is confirmed, the best place for the patient is CCU. Remember that streptokinase is contraindicated after surgery.

Chapter II.15

PULMONARY OEDEMA

Chapter II.15

PULMONARY OEDEMA

KEY POINTS

Pulmonary oedema is not uncommon after surgery. It may be
cardiogenic or non-cardiogenic.

Pulmonary oedema does not automatically imply fluid overload,
though this is an important cause.

Patients treated for **heart failure** are at special risk. Fluid overload, pain,
hypothermia or myocardial ischaemia can tip the balance. Most often
it is a combination of factors.

Cardiogenic pulmonary oedema is treated with oxygen, opiates,
diuretics and vasodilators. Non-cardiogenic pulmonary oedema
should be managed on ITU.

Introduction

Pulmonary oedema is an abnormal accumulation of fluid in the extravascular
spaces and tissues of the lung. It is not an uncommon cause of respiratory
distress in surgical patients.

Physiology

The factors that affect the movement of fluid in and out of the pulmonary
capillary were first described by Starling (see Figure II.15.1).

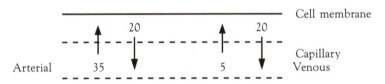

Figure II.15.1. Starling forces (mmHg).

Hydrostatic pressure forces fluid out of the capillary. This force is opposed
by colloid oncotic pressure, by virtue of the fact that the protein content of
interstitial fluid is much less than in the intravascular compartment.

At the arterial end: hydrostatic pressure is ~35 mmHg; colloid oncotic
pressure is ~20 mmHg and the net outward pressure is 15 mmHg.

At the venous end: hydrostatic pressure is ~5 mmHg; colloid oncotic pressure is ~20 mmHg and the net inward pressure is 15 mmHg.

Most fluid passes back into the capillary at the venous end, and the rest drains out via the lymphatics. If excessive fluid leaks from the capillary, pulmonary oedema results. This has two stages:

1. *Interstitial oedema*: characterized by engorgement of the interstitial space. The effects on lung function are subtle, though the lungs become stiffer and the patient usually complains of breathlessness. There are radiological changes (see Chapter II.17) but the condition may be difficult to detect.
2. *Alveolar oedema*: when fluid passes into the alveoli themselves. The effects of this are dramatic, with shrinking of alveoli, stiffer lungs, increased work of breathing and impaired gas exchange. The transition from interstitial to alveolar oedema tends to occur suddenly, for reasons that are not clearly understood (by us).

Mechanisms

There are three basic mechanisms which lead to increased fluid leak from capillaries:

1. Increased hydrostatic pressure in the capillary (e.g. in left ventricular failure).
2. Reduced colloid oncotic pressure (e.g. in hypoproteinaemia).
3. Increased capillary permeability (e.g. in aspiration pneumonitis or adult respiratory distress syndrome).

For the purposes of management, it is convenient to divide the causes of pulmonary oedema into cardiogenic and non-cardiogenic.

Cardiogenic pulmonary oedema

Presentation

History. Pulmonary oedema is most likely to occur in a patient with known ischaemic, hypertensive or rheumatic heart disease and may be associated with overenthusiastic fluid therapy. The patient complains of sudden, severe dyspnoea made worse on lying flat.

Examination. There may be tachycardia, sweating, cool peripheries, raised jugular venous pressure, gallop rhythm with a third heart sound ('KenTUCKy, KenTUCKy'). The blood pressure is often elevated, but hypotension is a grave finding indicative of cardiogenic shock, for which the management is different (see Chapter II.11). There are bilateral basal crepitations, and there may be an audible wheeze. Sputum is pink and frothy. Murmurs may be present, and a new murmur is a significant finding.

Investigations. The diagnosis of pulmonary oedema should be obvious clinically, and investigations are aimed more at finding a cause.

- Chest X-ray: the CXR findings are described in more detail in Chapter II.17, but note that a *normal* sized heart strongly suggests a non-cardiogenic cause.
- ECG should be done, looking for acute MI or dysrhythmia.
- Cardiac enzymes, in cases of suspected myocardial infarction. If the patient has recently had surgery, make sure to ask for CK-MB isoenzyme.

- Echocardiogram may be indicated to examine valve function, myocardial contractility and ejection fraction, as recommended by a cardiologist.
- CVP should not be required to make a diagnosis in the acute case. Readings will be higher than the 'normal' range, and should fall on treatment.
- Blood gases in severe cases where respiratory failure is suspected.

'Borderline cardiac failure'

This term is often used to describe patients with chronic heart disease who, whilst not in overt failure, are at risk of developing pulmonary oedema in certain circumstances. Such patients are particularly at risk in the perioperative period. Factors which may tip the balance are:

- Fluid overload. Patients with chronic heart failure cannot cope with as wide a range of filling pressures as a healthy patient, and aggressive fluid resuscitation can lead to pulmonary oedema. More commonly, however fear of this complication leads to a tendency to be excessively *miserly* with i.v. fluid.
- Systemic vasoconstriction, which acts by causing redistribution of fluid from systemic to pulmonary circulations, for example pain, hypothermia or the wearing-off of anaesthetic drugs.
- Myocardial ischaemia or infarction, and dysrhythmias.
  In most cases, there is a combination of factors that leads to deterioration.

Management

1. Sit up, give oxygen by mask (**not** 24%).
2. If there is evidence of cardiogenic shock (i.e. hypotension) or oliguria get help early.
3. Titrate in some i.v. narcotic (e.g. morphine 2 mg at 2-min intervals up to a maximum of 10 mg). This reduces venous tone, and alleviates agitation and anxiety.
4. Frusemide 20–40 mg i.v. The immediate effect of this drug is venodilation, which helps to offload the left ventricle. Later there is a diuresis.
   Note: this is the latest stage at which to ask for help. If the patient has improved, fine. If not, you should not proceed without senior assistance, for example a medical registrar.
5. Identify and treat dysrhythmias (see Chapter II.12).
6. Consider vasodilators for example isosorbide dinitrate ('Isoket') by i.v. infusion.
7. In severe cases with respiratory failure, ventilation on the ICU may be required.
8. Further measures are required for cardiogenic shock (hypotension, oliguria) or respiratory failure that results from pulmonary oedema. This may involve inotropes, invasive monitoring, ventilation, and one-to-one nursing. In other words, this is a job for ITU.

Non-cardiogenic pulmonary oedema

Causes

- Adult respiratory distress syndrome (ARDS). This is a final common pathway for a variety of major insults such as trauma, shock, sepsis, pancreatitis, burns, obstetric disasters or multiple organ failure. The basic mechanism is an increase in capillary permeability.

- Pulmonary aspiration of gastric contents (see Chapter II.17).
- Pneumonias and septicaemia.
- Allergic reactions to drugs or blood products.
- Neurogenic pulmonary oedema. This is a rare condition in which pulmonary oedema accompanies an acute intracranial lesion such as head injury, tumour or haemorrhage.

Diagnosis
The diagnosis of non-cardiogenic pulmonary oedema is suggested by an absence of specific features of cardiac failure. Normally this is obvious from the history alone, for example known chronic heart failure, or obvious precipitating cause such as pulmonary aspiration. In difficult cases, the diagnosis is suggested by pulmonary oedema in the presence of a normal-sized heart, or normal pulmonary capillary wedge pressure.

Management
Most cases of non-cardiogenic pulmonary oedema are managed on ITU. The specific management depends on the precise cause, but supportive management is likely to involve ventilation, optimization of filling pressures and maintenance of colloid oncotic pressure by avoidance of hypo-proteinaemia.

Chapter II.16

CARDIAC ARREST

CARDIAC ARREST

KEY POINTS

Know your hospital's DNR policy.
Keep your basic CPR skills up to at least the standard of the general
    public. Better still, do the ALS course.

The cardiac arrest team

Usually consists of a house physician, a medical SHO or registrar, and an
anaesthetist. In most hospitals, a senior nurse and a porter also carry an
arrest bleep. The medical registrar is 'in charge' of any arrest, and is
responsible for the direction of therapy.

Who to resuscitate?

Clearly there are circumstances where it would be inappropriate to perform
cardiopulmonary resuscitation (CPR), for example for terminally ill patients
where death is expected. Deciding which patients are appropriate for a 'Do
not resuscitate' (DNR) order is difficult, and serious problems have occurred
in the past. The issue has prompted directives from the Chief Medical
Officer and from medical and nursing professional bodies, who have
recommended that each hospital have a clearly documented and standardized
policy.

You are encouraged to become familiar with the policy of your own
hospital, but it is likely to be similar to the following:
- DNR is appropriate where CPR is unlikely to succeed, where it is
  contrary to the expressed wishes of a competent patient, or where CPR is
  likely to be followed by a length or quality of life which is unacceptable to
  the patient. DNR on the basis of age alone is not appropriate.
- The decision for a DNR order rests ultimately with the consultant in
  charge of the patient's care. He/she may choose to delegate this to other
  staff. Medical and nursing staff should be in agreement about any
  individual DNR order. The decision should be taken as soon as possible
  where arrest is deemed likely. The decision should be reviewed regularly.
- When a DNR order is taken, it should be documented clearly in the
  notes, and a brief rationale should be given. The senior nurse should be
  informed, and he/she should make appropriate documentation in the
  nursing notes.

Note that it is not necessary for the patient to be in arrest for an arrest to
be called. It is the quickest way to get senior help and should be used
whenever arrest is considered likely, for example dysrhythmia with
hypotension, bradycardia in an asthmatic, anaphylaxis.

DNR vs. withdrawal of treatment

This commonly causes confusion. It may be appropriate to continue various supportive measures in a patient who is the subject of a DNR order. It is justified to recognize that a patient's only chance lies in, for example, antibiotic therapy, and should this fail the chances of surviving an arrest are very slim. Treatment aimed at alleviating suffering should always be continued.

Basic life support

This skill is increasingly within the capabilities of members of the public, so there is no excuse for any doctor to be ignorant of basic CPR.
1. *Call for help.*
2. *Airway* look for response by shouting "are you alright". Open and maintain the airway with jaw thrust/chin lift and head extension.
3. *Breathing.* Listen at the lips whilst watching the chest. If there is no apparent respiratory effort or shifting of air, begin mouth to mouth, or mouth to mask resuscitation. Mouth to mask is best, if you have a Laerdal pocket mask handy, and it is more effective than an Ambu bag in inexperienced hands.
4. *Circulation.* Feel for a carotid pulse (for 5 sec). If absent, start external cardiac massage at a rate of 80/min. (For some reason, the word 'bedsprings' helps those learning CPR to get the frequency of compressions right. I can't think why.) Place one hand on top of the other, on the lower sternum, and give sharp compressions to depress the sternum by 3–4 cm each time. If alone, give 15 compressions for every two breaths.

Advanced life support

This is the continuation of basic life support. Intubation, ventilation by self-inflating bag or mechanical ventilator, and securing of i.v. access should be performed. An ECG monitor should be connected. For witnessed arrests, a pre-cordial thump is recommended, as this can sometimes restore cardiac output. Further treatment then depends upon the heart rhythm.

Ventricular fibrillation (VF) or pulseless VT:
    DC shock 200 J
    DC shock 200 J
    DC shock 360 J
    Adrenaline 1 mg i.v.
    Continue CPR
    DC shock 360 J
    DC shock 360 J
    DC shock 360 J
    Consider lignocaine 100 mg (= 5 ml of 2%) or bretylium
Asystole where VF cannot be excluded:
    DC shock 200 J
    DC shock 200 J
    DC shock 360 J
    then as for asystole (overleaf)

Asystole:

Adrenaline 1 mg i.v.

Continue CPR

Atropine 3 mg i.v. once only

Consider pacing

Electromechanical dissociation (QRS complexes with no output):

Differential diagnosis is hypovolaemia, tension pneumothorax, pulmonary embolism or cardiac tamponade. Consider specific therapy for each.

Adrenaline 1 mg i.v.

CPR

Repeat as required

When to give up

If a cardiac output is restored, the patient should be admitted to ITU for further management. The prognosis depends upon the underlying cause of the arrest, and the hypoxic interval, that is the length of time for which there was no output. The longer the hypoxic interval, the greater the chance of neurological damage. The arterial pH correlates fairly well with outcome: if pH >7.20, the outlook is reasonable. Survival where the post-arrest pH <7.0 is poor.

If an output is not restored, a decision has to be made on when to discontinue CPR. This is normally by consensus of those present, including nurses, with the final say given to the medical registrar. Normally, 20 min of unsuccessful resuscitation is considered enough. The situations where prolonged resuscitation is indicated are:

- Hypothermia: successful resuscitation without neurological damage is possible with severe hypothermia, even after extraordinary lengths of time. CPR should be continued until body temperature is normal. Rewarming may require cardiopulmonary bypass.
- Suspected drug overdose.
- Any arrest in children, who tend to have a better neurological prognosis than adults.

During prolonged resuscitation, adrenaline 1 mg is given every 5 min. Bicarbonate should only be given for severe acidosis (i.e. pH <7.0) as documented on blood gas analysis. Plenty of pairs of hands are required to share in the cardiac massage.

Chapter II.17

RESPIRATORY PROBLEMS

Chapter II.17

RESPIRATORY PROBLEMS

Effect of surgery and anaesthesia on respiratory function

There are four main effects:
1. Reduction of lung compliance. Stiffer lungs, in other words.
2. Ventilation/perfusion mismatch. Anaesthesia and surgery upset the delicate mechanisms that usually match perfusion to ventilation in the lung.
3. Hypoventilation. This has a variety of causes:
    - Central causes: from respiratory depressant effects of anaesthetic agents and opioids, or CNS pathology.
    - Peripheral causes: obesity, abdominal distension, tight dressings, pain, or any lung pathology which increases work of breathing (e.g. bronchospasm or sputum retention).
4. Ciliary dysfunction. Giving dry gas directly to the airway has a damaging effect on respiratory mucosa and ciliary function that persists into the postoperative period.

It is not surprising therefore, that a common finding after surgery is **hypoxaemia**. It is worse in the presence of chronic lung disease, but the site and scale of the operation, and the patient's age, are also important factors.

> *Dips of oxygen saturation to* **<50%** *are commonplace after major abdominal surgery. Episodic hypoxaemia occurs especially at night, within 72 h of the operation. It is known that this hypoxia is associated with episodes of severe myocardial ischaemia.*

As the house surgeon, you have a useful role in keeping your patients pink:
- Identify and pay attention to those at risk: abdominal or thoracic surgery, elderly, smokers, 'cronnie-bronnies'.
- Prescribe oxygen therapy. (Yes, write it on the drug chart – see below.)
- Ensure good analgesia (see below and Chapters II.1–II.4).

Oxygen therapy

The mainstay of management of postoperative pulmonary problems is oxygen therapy. It is grossly underused.

Methods
Standard facemask ('Hudson' mask). This is the commonest method. Oxygen is passed through a tube to a simple mask, where it is mixed with inspired air drawn through large holes. Oxygen can be humidified before delivery. The mask cannot deliver very high concentrations of oxygen, and the exact inspired oxygen concentration depends on the *pattern* of breathing. If the patient takes rapid, sharp breaths with a high peak inspiratory flow-rate, the inspired oxygen concentration will be similar to that of air, whereas if the patient takes slow shallow breaths, the inspired oxygen concentration may rise.

These masks are also called variable performance masks because it impossible to tell what the true inspired oxygen concentration is. Unless you forget to turn the oxygen on.

High airflow oxygen enrichment (HAFOE) masks (e.g. Ventimasks®). These masks get over the problem of variable inspired oxygen concentration by applying the Venturi principle. A jet of oxygen is passed through a short aperture in the mask where it entrains a fixed proportion of air. The result is a flow of gas with a known oxygen concentration at about 50 litres per minute. Provided the patient's peak inspiratory flow-rate is less than this (it usually is), the inspired oxygen concentration will be the same. The masks come in a selection of concentrations, usually 24%, 28% and 35%, and are the preferred delivery method for patients with significant chronic lung disease. The masks can be identified by the concentration marking on the hub.

Notice that the highest concentration you can give with a HAFOE mask is 35%, so if you need more than this, use a different system.

Reservoir bag masks. The reservoir bag fills with oxygen during expiration, and the patient empties it during inspiration. It is claimed that these masks can deliver 85% oxygen. They tend to be used for trauma, and can usually be found in A&E.

Nasal cannulae. These are fine tubes which are placed below the patient's nostrils, then threaded over the ears like a pair of spectacles. Their main advantage is comfort, and patients can usually be persuaded to wear them for long periods. Video surveillance studies have shown that patients rarely keep facemasks on continuously. However, nasal cannulae cannot give high concentrations of oxygen and are not suitable for very sick patients.

Complications of oxygen therapy

Respiratory depression. There is a common reluctance amongst doctors to give oxygen to anyone with the slightest evidence of chronic obstructive airways disease. "Oxygen is a drug" we are told. "We must be careful". It is the fear of this **rare** complication that results in the withholding of oxygen from hundreds of thousands of hypoxaemic patients. It's true, oxygen *is* a drug – an extremely safe and effective one.

There is a group of patients, who represent only a small subset of those with chronic lung disease, that maintain grossly abnormal blood gases. As a result of long-standing lung damage, they have chronically increased work of breathing, and hypoventilate to the extent that the central chemoreceptors become tolerant of very high levels of P_aCO_2. Their kidneys compensate for the respiratory acidosis by retaining bicarbonate, so the arterial pH is about normal. Instead, these patients rely on *hypoxia* for respiratory drive.

If such a patient is given an excessive concentration of oxygen, particularly in times of crisis, P_aO_2 may rise, and respiratory drive will be lost. This causes progressive respiratory depression, and increasing P_aCO_2. In excess, CO_2 causes progressive depression of consciousness and eventually apnoea. Once the patient stops breathing, hypoxia returns, but it is not adequate to overcome the depressive effects of the huge CO_2 levels, and unless the patient receives mechanical ventilation, he dies.

Remember hypoxic drive is **rare**. If you think your patient may have hypoxic drive, they may still benefit from oxygen therapy, but it must be given in a controlled manner. Ventimasks are the delivery method of choice, as standard Hudson masks can be dangerous.

How to identify a patient with 'hypoxic drive'

The end of the bed: the sort of patients we are talking about are *bright blue*.

History: long history of chronic lung disease. Shortness of breath at rest or minimal exertion. Bronchospasm, chronic purulent cough (cigarette smoking alone is *not* a predictor). These patients are very difficult to anaesthetize safely. Previous uneventful general anaesthesia makes hypoxic drive *extremely unlikely*.

Examination: cyanosis and asterixis (flapping tremor).

Investigations: blood gases: low P_aO_2 (<75 mmHg), high P_aCO_2 (>55 mmHg) *and* slightly low or normal pH under normal circumstances breathing air. Look through any old notes to find previous blood gas measurements. Some U&E results give a bicarbonate level. Be suspicious if bicarbonate is >30 mmol/l.

Controlled oxygen therapy means giving progressively increased concentrations of oxygen, and at each step measuring blood gases after 10 min or so. If you see an increase in P_aO_2 without an increase in P_aCO_2, it is safe to proceed to the next concentration up. If you see an increase in P_aCO_2, go back down to the step before, and *prescribe* this much oxygen on the patient's drug chart. Don't write it in the PRN section.

The other complications of oxygen therapy are pretty small print stuff:

- *Oxygen toxicity* is seen in laboratory animals, and may or may not occur in humans. It is said to occur if concentrations of >60% are inhaled for long periods (i.e. > 24 h). Hypoxia should *never* be tolerated because of fear of oxygen toxicity.
- *Retrolental fibroplasia* is a condition seen in neonates who are ventilated with high oxygen concentrations, causing fibrosis behind the lens of the eye, and blindness.
- *Blowing your house up* is a condition seen sometimes in inveterate old smokers on domiciliary oxygen, who can't resist one last fag for old time's sake. Oxygen, as you know, strongly supports combustion.

Indications for oxygen therapy

1. *Cyanosis* or documented hypoxaemia as measured by pulse oximetry
2. *Major surgery.* For 24 h postoperatively, and at night for 3 nights.
3. *Shock and severe haemorrhage.* Any cause of shock results in a reduction of oxygen delivery.
4. *Myocardial ischaemia* or those at risk of it (see Chapter II.14).
5. *Conditions of high metabolic rate.* For example, fever, rigors, thyroid crisis, malignant hyperpyrexia.
6. *Reduced consciousness or hypoventilation.*

Analgesia and respiratory dysfunction

Postoperative analgesia in respiratory disease deserves particular attention. Inadequate analgesia is unpleasant and unacceptable for any patient but, for those with pre-existing respiratory disease, it can be disastrous. Any source of pain which prevents movement, deep breathing or coughing will hamper a patient's ability to clear secretions from the lungs. The resulting immobility and sputum retention is a potent recipe for respiratory infection, which may lead to respiratory failure, and even death. Any operative wound in the chest or abdomen may cause enough pain to affect coughing, and the nearer it is to the diaphragm, the worse the effect. Even painful wounds in the extremities can upset respiration by causing tachypnoea, anxiety or bronchospasm.

On the other hand, excessive or ill-chosen analgesic regimens can have an equally catastrophic effect. All opioids have respiratory-depressant properties, and excessive doses can be dangerous in decompensated patients. In addition, many drugs, including some opioids, can worsen bronchospasm in susceptible individuals.

For this group of patients, therefore, there is a fine line between respiratory failure caused by action, and respiratory failure caused by neglect. The following is a guide to the various techniques available. For more detail on postoperative analgesia, see Chapters II.1–II.4.

Epidural analgesia

This is definitely the gold standard in this situation. A well-functioning epidural can provide the most effective pain relief available, in many cases allowing movement and coughing without pain. In addition, the respiratory side-effects are comparatively trivial: a dense block may affect intercostal muscle function, and there is a reported incidence of respiratory depression when opioids are used, but there is growing evidence that the importance of the latter has been overestimated. An anaesthetist is required to place the catheter, and the patient should be nursed in a high dependency area afterwards.

Intravenous opioids
The name of the game here is titration. The best way to match dose with requirement is to let the patient do it himself, with a patient-controlled analgesia device (PCA). If a PCA is not available, an infusion may work reasonably well, provided a carefully titrated loading dose is given before the infusion is started. For patients with reversible airways disease, pethidine or fentanyl are preferred over morphine, diamorphine or papaveretum, all of which may worsen bronchospasm.

Opioids by other routes
Intermittent i.m. injection should be avoided at all costs in these patients, except for short-lived pain in mild disease. Don't be fooled by the supposedly 'safer' opioids such as codeine and its derivatives. All opioids, contrary to the claims of some manufacturers, cause respiratory depression in direct proportion to their analgesic potency. If they don't affect respiration, it's because they don't work.

Peripheral nerve blocks
Occasionally, surgical pain, particularly in the peripheries, is amenable to treatment with continuous peripheral nerve block. Examples are axillary brachial plexus block for arm wounds, and femoral nerve blocks for pain in the upper leg. These have the advantage of providing excellent pain relief without the risk of respiratory depression, and allow the avoidance of opioids.

Non-steroidal anti-inflammatory drugs
NSAIDS are effective adjuncts to postoperative pain management, and reduce the requirement for opioids. Unfortunately, the fly in this particular ointment is the significant incidence of bronchospasm after their use. The effect is often delayed, and there is a significant incidence of even mild asthma sufferers being hospitalized with severe exacerbations several days after taking an NSAID.

Although not all chest sufferers have reversible airways disease and, of those that do, not all are sensitive to NSAIDs, it is difficult to identify those at risk. The sensible advice therefore is to avoid them unless a patient has taken an NSAID without difficulty many times before.

Sputum control

The ability to effectively clear secretions can be a matter of life or death for chest patients (or anyone, for that manner). General measures to assist this process include humidified oxygen therapy, good general hydration (though overhydration is bad), and pain relief sufficient to allow good coughing. Physiotherapy is the mainstay of treatment, including percussion and postural drainage.

Physiotherapists have an extremely important role in perioperative management of chest patients, and it is worth consulting them early. As well as assisting with sputum clearance, they can instruct the patient with deep breathing techniques (such as incentive spirometry) and general rehabilitation.

Respiratory distress

When called to a patient with respiratory distress, there is a fairly clearly defined differential diagnosis:
- Asthma.
- Pneumonia, collapse, consolidation.
- Pulmonary oedema.
- Pulmonary embolus.
- Pneumothorax.
- Pulmonary aspiration.
- Pleural effusions.

Asthma and bronchospasm
Worsening asthma is heralded by dyspnoea, audible wheeze and use of accessory muscles. There are five important danger signs which signify a severe episode and poor prognosis. Assistance from ITU and/or respiratory medicine should be sought if any of the following is present:
- Tachycardia >120 (though this is most often caused by treatment with β-2 agonists or theophylline. If HR <60 in acute asthma, call the cardiac arrest team).
- Inability to speak.
- Silent chest (signifies severe hypoventilation).
- Cyanosis or SaO_2 <93%.
- Depressed consciousness.

All patients with worsening asthma should have a chest X-ray to exclude pneumothorax, respiratory infection or aspiration. A set of blood gases should be drawn. Please note that a P_aCO_2 in the *normal range* is bad, suggesting impending deterioration. Patients with acute asthma who are coping well usually hyperventilate, with a P_aCO_2 of 25–30 mmHg.

Management should include humidified oxygen, salbutamol and ipratropium by nebulizer, and i.v. steroids (e.g. 200 mg hydrocortisone 6-hourly for an average adult). The quantity of nebulized bronchodilator that reaches the lower airways in acute asthma is small, and if a single nebulizer has limited effect it should be followed immediately by another, then another. Each nebulizer then becomes progressively more effective. Four-hourly nebulizers are for maintenance, not emergency management.

If these measures fail to bring about an improvement, or if the patient continues to deteriorate clinically, as demonstrated by a rising P_aCO_2, then this is definitely time to call for help. Further measures, like the use of aminophylline should be undertaken only with senior assistance.

Sedatives are *absolutely* contraindicated. Opioids should also be avoided if at all possible, and anaesthetic assistance should be sought if severe pain co-exists.

Pneumonia, collapse, consolidation
Hospital-acquired pneumonia occurs in 0.5–5% of all in-patients, and 10–40% of those on ICU. The commonest causative organism is *Strep. pneumoniae*, but Gram-negative organisms are seen more often than they are

in community-acquired pneumonias, and 10–20% of infections are caused by more than one organism. Diagnosis, suggested by cough, fever, purulent sputum and consolidation on chest X-ray, should be confirmed by blood cultures (see Chapter II.19).

Sputum clearance is even more important than antibiotic therapy. Involve the physiotherapist early.

Patients commonly develop lobar collapse or atelectasis after surgery, and this is a frequent cause of hypoxaemia. It is readily identified on X-ray (see below). Again, analgesia, sputum clearance and oxygen therapy are the mainstay of management.

Pulmonary oedema
A detailed account of pulmonary oedema appears in Chapter II.15, but suffice it to say that pulmonary oedema is a potent cause of respiratory distress, hypoxaemia and ventilatory failure.

Pulmonary embolus
Embolic phenomena account for a significant proportion of cases of respiratory distress and sudden death, and *any* patient laid up in bed after surgery is at risk. Special risk factors are dealt with in Chapter II.23. There are few conditions whose presence (or *perceived* presence) cause more dilemmas and lost sleep for young doctors.

Of PEs, 40–60% are asymptomatic; 10% are fatal. The common signs are non-specific, and the specific signs are rare, though pulmonary embolus should always feature in your differential diagnosis of respiratory distress.

In the dyspnoeic patient in the small hours, it is a diagnosis of *exclusion*. Clinical features are:

Symptoms.
- Dyspnoea: common. Sudden onset breathlessness is the most reliable indicator.
- Syncope: occasionally.
- Pleuritic chest pain and haemoptysis: this occurs in pulmonary *infarction*, which is only rarely a consequence of PE.
- Palpitations: AF can occur if there is pre-existing cardiac disease.

Signs.
- Tachycardia and tachypnoea: common.
- Low grade fever: may occur.
- Wheeze: sometimes.
- Hypotension common in massive PE.

Investigations.
- CXR: minimal change. May be some loss of volume. Infarction (with the classic 'wedge' appearance) and pleural effusion are *rare*.
- ECG: sinus tachycardia is the usual finding. Acute-onset AF may be seen. '$S_1 Q_3 T_3$', right axis deviation and RV ischaemia are *rare*.
- Blood gases: may show reduced P_aO_2 but not always. P_aCO_2 usually low.
- Scans: perfusion scan can exclude, V/Q scan required for definitive proof of diagnosis.

From this you can see that most patients with a PE will be dyspnoeic, tachycardic, with normal CXR and sinus tachycardia on the ECG, and have no other signs. The diagnosis cannot be confirmed at night, and you have to decide whether or not to heparinize.

The first thing to do is exclude other causes: pulmonary oedema, pneumothorax, pulmonary collapse, consolidation, aspiration. If there are no other likely causes, then a PE can be presumed, and a request for V/Q scan should be made at the next opportunity. Many hospitals do perfusion scans every day, but may only do a full V/Q scan once a week. This is because the isotope used for the ventilation part of the scan has a very short half-life. A normal perfusion scan can exclude a pulmonary embolus.

In the meantime, however, there is the question of whether to anti-coagulate. It could be argued that once the diagnosis is made, however tentatively, then this should be followed up with heparin therapy. Certainly it would be difficult to defend yourself if the patient died of another pulmonary embolus in the meantime, and you didn't treat.

On the other hand, anticoagulation carries potential hazards of its own, especially in patients who have had certain forms of surgery. The safest approach is to present your findings to your next on-call, to make sure that there is no particular contraindication to heparinization. If not, give 5000 units i.v., followed by an infusion of 20 000–24 000 units per day.

Monitor the clotting times regularly. An APTT of 2–3 times control is required. If the clotting times fall below this, it is usually necessary to give a small bolus (e.g. 2000 units) *as well as* increasing the infusion rate. If the diagnosis is confirmed with a scan, treatment with warfarin will be required for 3–6 months. When starting warfarin, remember its interactions, particularly with NSAIDs.

Pneumothorax
This can be spontaneous, trauma-related or iatrogenic.
1. Spontaneous pneumothoraces occur in tall, young skinny males, or those with chronic obstructive airways disease or asthma.
2. Trauma-related pneumothoraces normally occur as a result of rib fractures or penetrating chest wounds.
3. Iatrogenic pneumothoraces are perhaps the most common in the perioperative period. A number of procedures carry a risk of pleural puncture, and often the pneumothorax does not develop until several hours later. The commonest are:
   - central line insertion, by subclavian or internal jugular routes;
   - some forms of brachial plexus block;
   - as a result of some forms of surgery (e.g. nephrectomy).

An index of suspicion with a breathless patient is the most important weapon. The diagnosis is readily confirmed on an upright chest X-ray. Management of a large pneumothorax is with a chest drain. Small non-traumatic ones can sometimes be managed by aspiration, or 'watched' with serial chest X-rays. A physician can advise.

Pulmonary aspiration
This is a clinical syndrome resulting from inhalation of gastric contents. Predisposing factors include anaesthesia, particularly for emergency surgery, depressed consciousness, disorders of swallowing or cough, use of nasogastric tubes, pregnancy and tracheostomy. It presents with dyspnoea,

wheezing, cough and rhonchi, usually within 2 h of the episode. In severe cases there is cyanosis, tachycardia and hypotension. The diagnosis is often difficult to prove, unless gastric contents are visibly suctioned from the trachea. Chest X-ray changes include multilobar infiltrates which can be alveolar or interstitial, and may be unilateral. Occasionally, frank pulmonary oedema is seen. Management is supportive: humidified oxygen, hydration, and artificial ventilation if respiratory failure supervenes. Antibiotics are recommended only if there is definite evidence for infection, when they are usually aimed at Gram-negative organisms. Steroids are no longer recommended, and probably worsen the outcome.

Pleural effusions
Pleural effusions have numerous causes, and it is beyond the scope of this book to list and explain them all. There are instances, however, where a pleural effusion causes (or more likely, contributes to) postoperative respiratory dysfunction. Remember, an effusion you can see on a chest X-ray is at least 150 ml, and one you can pick up clinically is likely to be huge. Needle drainage (preferably with ultrasound guidance) is indicated where respiratory function is borderline.

The emergency chest X-ray

Nearly all the X-rays you order at night will be the AP portable kind.

It is very difficult to take good quality films of crumpled foaming-at-the-mouth octogenarians under these circumstances, but usually the question being asked of the film is simple (e.g. "how many lungs?"), not difficult ("is there type IIIa pulmonary Von Skrotum's disease?"). The conditions that can be diagnosed with relative ease on all but the most dreadful X-rays are:
- pulmonary oedema;
- lobar collapse;
- consolidation;
- pleural effusion;
- pneumothorax;
...and these are the very things that will most often feature in your differential diagnosis.

Collapse (atelectasis)
This is a very common cause of hypoxia in the postoperative period, when it is usually caused by mucous plugging. It may affect any lobe and be partial or complete, depending on how much air remains in it. The general signs are:
- Increased opacity of the affected lobe. Remember, however, that the collapsed lung tissue may be obscured by other structures, especially the heart.
- Loss of volume. This is an extremely important sign and can be spotted on all but the worst films. The three main changes seen are raised hemidiaphragm, shift of the mediastinal structures towards the lesion, and crowding of ribs on the affected side.
- Hyperlucency of adjacent unaffected lobes is sometimes seen, as they hyperexpand to help fill the space left by the collapse.

In addition, the collapse of individual lobes causes characteristic patterns on the chest X-ray (Figure II.17.1). Remember that the collapsed lung may be obscured and the only clue will be fairly obvious loss of volume.

Examination of an emergency chest X-ray

First of all look at the film's quality:

1. Is it rotated? The tips of the clavicles should be equidistant from the vertebral column. Rotation will affect the appearance of mediastinal shift, an important sign.
2. Is it correctly penetrated? On a good film, the thoracic vertebral bodies should be just about visible behind the heart. This becomes important when assessing the lung fields for shadowing.
3. Is it erect or supine? Supine films make diagnosis of pleural effusion or pneumothorax more difficult.

Next, systematically examine the film for abnormalities. A simple system is as follows:

- Mediastinum and heart. Position: trachea should be central, one-third of the heart should be to the right of the midline.
  Borders: the silhouette should be sharp. Loss of any border may suggest adjacent lobar collapse. Heart size and mediastinal width are difficult to assess on an AP film, but gross changes can be detected.
- Soft tissue and bone. Look at ribs carefully for fractures, and compare the spacing on each side. Don't get caught out by apparent hyperlucency of one lung caused by mastectomy, or loss of pectoralis muscle on one side.
- Lung fields. Lucency: compare corresponding zones, left to right, they should be similar. If there is shadowing, does it correspond to a particular lobe?
- Diaphragm: the mid-point of the right hemidiaphragm should be at the level of the anterior 5th–7th ribs. The left is usually 2–3 cm lower. One raised hemidiaphragm suggests loss of volume. If they are both raised it is probably due to poor inspiration. Costophrenic angles should be sharp.
- Vascular markings: are they visible right to the edges? (if not, consider pneumothorax) are they more visible in the upper lobes? (this is indicative of cardiac failure).
- Pleura, hila, etc.: many things can be said about the pleural thickness, etc., but not at 3 a.m.

Consolidation
This is an area of homogeneous increased radio-opacity. It can be any size. The main features are:
- ill-defined margins;
- irregular shape;
- *no* loss of volume (i.e. no mediastinal shift, no raised hemidiaphragm, no rib crowding);
- air bronchogram is common. This is seen when the bronchi become clearly visible against an opaque 'ground glass' background.

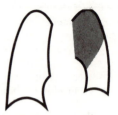

Left upper lobe collapse

The upper lobe is actually anterior to most of the lower lobe on the left, and collapses to a hazy 'veil-like' appearance. Notice the loss of the left mediastinal border

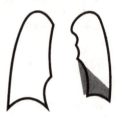

Left lower lobe collapse

The appearance is seen when the lobe is partially collapsed. Note the preservation of the left heart border. When fully collapsed, the lobe hides behind the heart. In this case, all that is seen is the loss of volume and a double left-sided heart border

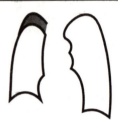

Right upper lobe collapse

The lobe collapses to a triangle upwards and medially. The lesser fissure is displaced upwards, and may be convex, as shown. The right upper mediastinal shadow is lost

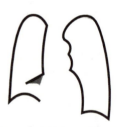

Right middle lobe collapse

The fissure is pulled downwards and there may only be a subtle shadowing. The biggest clue is the loss of the right heart border

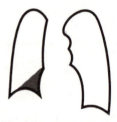

Right lower lobe collapse

This is the picture of partial collapse. Notice that the right heart border and diaphragm are preserved. As with left lower lobe, when completely collapsed, the lung fields may seem clear, and all that is seen is loss of volume and double right heart border

Figure II.17.1. Lobar collapse.

Pneumonia

The classical picture of community-acquired 'lobar' pneumonia, where *Strep. pneumoniae* is the commonest organism, is uniform consolidation in a single lobe. An air bronchogram is usually seen, and there is no loss of volume. However, pneumonias acquired in the pus factories we call 'hospitals' are often caused by Gram-negative agents or *Staph. aureus*, and the X-ray appearance may be different. Sometimes referred to as 'bronchopneumonia', it is seen as *patchy* segmental consolidation, which may be bilateral and predominantly affects the lower lobes. An air bronchogram is rarely seen, and there may be loss of volume.

Pneumothorax

There are two findings which are required for the diagnosis of pneumothorax: loss of vascular markings at the apex and laterally, **and** a visible lung edge. On a supine film the air collects anteriorly, it is more difficult to spot, but clues are a unilaterally lucent lung, or a translucent band parallel to the mediastinum or diaphragm. A tension pneumothorax is seen when mediastinal structures are displaced to the opposite side. Ideally, however, such an X-ray should not exist, as this is a clinical diagnosis, and must be treated immediately.

Pleural effusion

A large pleural effusion (300–500 ml) should be easy to detect on an erect chest film. The signs are a homogeneous opacification of the lower chest, with loss of costophrenic angle and hemidiaphragm. The upper margin is concave upwards, and is higher laterally than medially. The signs of small pleural effusion are easy to miss, but usually include loss of costophrenic angle.

Pulmonary oedema

Pulmonary oedema is basically an excess of fluid in the lungs that isn't in the intravascular compartment. Initially, the fluid is contained in the interstitial space and, as it worsens, it eventually spills into the alveolar air spaces. Interstitial oedema and alveolar oedema have different X-ray appearances. The signs are as follows:

- Interstitial oedema. *Septal lines.* Fluid collects in the interlobular septa. This is visible as short, horizontal lines 3–6 cm long, known as Kerley 'B' lines. They are best seen in the peripheral lower zones.
  Peribronchial cuffing. On normal X-rays, a few bronchi can be seen end-on in the hilar regions. In interstitial oedema their walls appear thickened
  Vascular changes. Vessel shadows are seen more clearly in the upper zones than lower, referred to as upper lobe blood diversion.
- Alveolar oedema. *Irregular shadowing.* Grey fluffy shadows are seen, more frequently in the lower zones. As it progresses, the shadows become confluent and whiter. Sometimes the hilar zones are more affected with sparing of the peripheries, giving a 'bat's wings' appearance. Eventually there is a total 'whiteout', with loss of any visible vascular markings.
  Pleural effusions. Commonly bilateral, but if unilateral it is more common on the right. Fluid may be seen in the horizontal fissure.
  Air bronchogram is common.

Respiratory failure and ventilation

When viewed at its simplest, the lung has basically two jobs: taking up oxygen and getting rid of carbon dioxide. When the lungs fail to work, therefore, they may fail to perform one or other of these tasks. Because of this, some bright spark decided that there should be two types of respiratory failure: type I, in which there is a problem with oxygen uptake, and type II, where there is a problem excreting carbon dioxide. It may not have escaped the brighter students that if you stop breathing, you get into both kinds of failure pretty quick, so yes, there is also the concept of *mixed* respiratory failure.

In the vast majority of cases, respiratory failure seen after surgery is the mixed variety, resulting from both poor oxygenation and increased work of breathing, leading eventually to hypoventilation. Whereas many measures can help to prevent the onset of failure, there is but one treatment: intermittent positive pressure ventilation (IPPV).

The benefits of IPPV in the exhausted, hypoxic, hypercapnic patient are numerous. Firstly, it provides adequate ventilation to control P_aCO_2 and, in doing so, removes all work of breathing. This reduces oxygen demand. In addition, by connecting the patient to a closed breathing system, high oxygen concentrations can be delivered, and positive end-expiratory pressure (PEEP) can be applied. This technique, whereby a small pressure (of usually ~5 cmH_2O) is maintained between ventilator breaths, improves oxygenation by increasing functional residual capacity (FRC) and reducing shunt (blood passing through unventilated areas of lung). Suctioning of secretions will benefit the patient who is too weak to cough.

Chapter II.18

OLIGURIA AND CATHETERS

OLIGURIA AND CATHETERS

KEY POINTS

Postoperative oliguria is nearly always due to hypovolaemia.
Fluid challenges are the mainstay of management, guided by repeated estimation of volume status and sometimes CVP.
Diuretics are usually harmful in this situation.
Acute renal failure is suggested by oliguria despite adequate fluid loading.

Introduction

A low urine output in the surgical patient is an important sign of hypovolaemia and may precede acute renal failure (ARF). This sign must never be ignored as ARF carries a significant mortality and is preventable in most cases. A urine volume of at least 0.5 ml/kg/h (1.0 ml/kg/h in children) is desirable in surgical patients. A volume of less than 20 ml/h is incompatible with minimum excretion of solute load, and below this volume accumulation of metabolites (urea, potassium, acid) will inevitably occur.

Detection

You can't diagnose oliguria unless you measure the urine output. Catheterize all high risk patients and use a buretted collection system. Those at high risk are:

Patient factors	Surgical factors
Diabetics	Major trauma, crush injuries
Chronic renal impairment	Burns, electrocutions
Jaundice	Hypovolaemia, hypoxia
Old age	Sepsis
Cardiac failure	Major abdominal cases
Severe connective tissue diseases	Major vascular cases
	Cardiac surgery

Baseline tests of renal function are also compulsory in these groups. Chronic renal impairment is suggested by a high creatinine (normal range 44–124 micromol/l) or high urea (2.5–6.6 mmol/l), and in worse cases by a metabolic acidosis and hyperkalaemia. All results have to be interpreted with a knowledge of the clinical picture. For instance, urea may be raised by dehydration, or potassium by spironolactone. Creatinine levels reflect total protein turnover, therefore a high serum creatinine is indicative of more severe disease in a frail elderly patient than in a young body-builder. More specialized tests of renal function, such as creatinine clearance, are not generally relevant to the surgical patient.

Management of oliguria

Start with a clinical examination, paying attention to the state of hydration (pulse, BP, mental state, skin turgor, eye turgor, dry mouth). Always consider the possibility of urinary retention or obstruction and examine for a full bladder; remember retention is a common cause of postoperative confusion. Exclude any signs of heart failure or fluid overload. The presence of peripheral oedema does not exclude the possibility of hypovolaemia; it may mean that your patient is having difficulty in distributing water correctly (see Chapter II.6).

You need to re-assess the effects of your interventions, so catheterize the patient if not done previously and arrange for hourly urine measurements.

The role of fluids

The smartest physician is dumber than the dumbest nephron. Virtually all cases of oliguria are the physiological response of the kidney to dehydration or hypovolaemia. Therefore, the reaction of the physician should be to correct the fluid deficit. A fluid challenge (e.g. 200 ml of a gelatin solution) is given over a short time and then the patient is completely reviewed. The process of assessment–treatment–reassessment is the key to success.

An improvement in vital signs and urine output confirms that your initial diagnosis of hypovolaemia was correct.

If there is no initial improvement in urine output, repeat the challenge. If oliguria persists you will need a more accurate way of assessing the patient's volume status, although your suspicion is still of hypovolaemia. A central line is indicated to measure CVP (central venous pressure). Remember that single readings are of little value; you need to make serial measurements to see what difference fluid challenges make. Provided the initial measurement is not grossly elevated (i.e. <15 cmH$_2$O), it is reasonable to give fluid challenges until either urine flow improves, or until you have elevated the CVP by 5 cmH$_2$O. If, despite this, urine output remains inadequate, you need to consider the possibility of ARF (see below). If the CVP is low (i.e. <5 cmH$_2$O) continue with fluid challenges. There is no such thing as a 'normal' CVP. The correct CVP for an individual patient is the value that results in an acceptable urine output and vital signs.

The role of diuretics

A dumb physician is much, much dumber than the dumbest nephron. When a kidney is working flat out to preserve water for its hypovolaemic owner, the worst thing you can do is to prevent it from doing its job by poisoning it with frusemide. Diuretics in this situation will worsen the hypovolaemia and increase the risk of ARF.

Diuretics can only be used safely when there is accurate knowledge of *volume status*, and usually this means under guidance of CVP readings in a high dependency unit.

The role of inotropes
If volume status has been normalized and the urine output remains low, a low dose of dopamine is often used (2.5 mcg/kg/min). This has diuretic, inotropic and (possibly) renal protective actions. This can usually be managed on a general surgical ward, but must have a high level of cardiovascular monitoring, including CVP.

General care
The kidney is put at increased risk by hypoxia, so oliguric patients should receive oxygen. Be sure to review the drug chart for any nephrotoxic drugs (aminoglycosides, NSAIDs, diuretics).

Making the diagnosis of ARF

As mentioned above, ARF is suspected when oliguria persists despite adequate CVP and blood pressure. A less common form is non-oliguric ARF, in which large volumes of dilute urine are formed. The diagnosis of ARF is confirmed by tests of blood and urine chemistry. The colour of the urine is of no value in assessing renal function.

In ARF the kidney loses its ability to concentrate the urine and to conserve sodium. Therefore a dilute urine is produced with an abnormally high sodium content. The following features differentiate ARF from a normal response to hypovolaemia:

Acute renal failure	Normal response to hypovolaemia
Dilute urine, variable volume	Concentrated urine, low volume
Iso-osmotic with plasma (290 mOsmol/l)	>500 mOsmol/l, specific gravity >1.016
High sodium content (>35 mmol/l)	Low sodium content (<20 mmol/l)
Low urine:plasma urea ratio (<3:1)	High urine:plasma urea ratio (>10:1)
Low urine urea content (<185 mmol/l)	

Later, uraemia, hyperkalaemia and a metabolic acidosis develop.

Referral
All cases of ARF should be referred either to ITU or to a renal HDU as the prognosis is improved enormously by expert care and renal replacement therapy. Urgent haemofiltration or haemodialysis is indicated for progressive hyperkalaemia, uraemia, acidosis and fluid overload.

Catheters

The indications for catheterization are as follows:
- for accurate measurement of urine output;
- in the management of acute retention;
- where normal micturition is difficult or impossible (e.g. spinal cord injury, major trauma, coma);
- for bladder irrigation (e.g. after prostate surgery).

Urethral catheters

Uretheral catheters are the commonest type. Significant problems can arise from trauma to the urethra, and bacteraemia. Points to remember:

- Analgesia: lignocaine jelly takes a while to work, and inadequate analgesia is probably the commonest reason for difficulty in passing a catheter in males. For best results, instil the jelly and hold it in with a penis clamp. Go away and have a cup of tea, then return and pass the catheter.
- Antisepsis: lignocaine jelly with chlorhexidine will reduce the bacteraemia produced by insertion. Many hospitals have agreed protocols for antibiotic cover of catheter insertion. This becomes especially important after orthopaedic implant surgery.
- Do **not** use wire introducers, or catheters with stiffened ends. These weapons are for experts only, and in inexperienced hands they can cause devastating urethral damage. If you have trouble passing an ordinary catheter **get help**.
- Take the weight off the bladder neck by taping the catheter to the leg.
- If you must clamp the catheter, do it distal to the insertion of the inflation channel. Clamping the inflation channel may permanently occlude it, rendering you unable to deflate the balloon. If you can't deflate the balloon, get help. Don't cut the end off.
- Don't forget to put the foreskin back into position after catheterizing males.

Suprapubic catheterization

Learn how to insert a suprapubic catheter. They are much preferred for the management of acute retention, as they avoid trauma to the urethra, probably lead to less sepsis, and considerably simplify the process of 'trial without catheter'. There are three contraindications:

1. *Absence of distended bladder.* The technique of insertion involves infiltration with local anaesthetic down through the bladder wall. You should never insert one unless you have aspirated urine.
2. *Post-TURP.*
3. *In patients with bladder tumours.*

Catheter problems

Blocking

Catheters occasionally become occluded, either from blood clots in haematuria, or from silt or crystalline matter. Assuming that the catheter did, at some stage, drain urine, the first move is to unblock it with a bladder syringe and some saline. If this is successful, it should be followed by a thorough bladder washout, involving the forceful instilling and drainage of several syringe-fulls of saline. If you are unable to clear the blockage, you may need to change the catheter.

Leaking around the catheter

This occasionally occurs when the lumen of the catheter is blocked (see above), but is most often the result of detrusor instability. The solution to this problem, although seemingly illogical, is to change the catheter for a size *smaller*.

Acute retention

This is common following major surgery, especially in men where it is usually associated with prostatic enlargement. Epidural analgesia increases the incidence. Sometimes a hot bath can relieve retention, but usually the treatment is catheterization. Remember:

- suprapubic is preferable to urethral;
- catheterize for painful retention **only**. Painless distension of the bladder is a chronic condition, which does not require catherization. The exception is retention with epidural analgesia, where the epidural may mask the pain.

Chapter II.19

FEVER

Chapter II.19

FEVER

Causes

'Normal' postoperative pyrexia

It is not uncommon for the stress of surgery to cause a low-grade pyrexia of 37.0–37.5°C. For this reason, it is not usually necessary to investigate and treat every fever in the early postoperative period in otherwise healthy patients.

Non-septic causes

Deep vein thrombosis, blood transfusion reactions and malignant hyperpyrexia all cause fevers in the absence of sepsis.

Septic causes

Obviously the most important group. The commonest sites of infection are:

1. *Chest.* Anaesthesia and surgery make the lungs stiffer and impair sputum clearance, a good recipe for chest infection. The commonest culprit is still *Strep. pneumoniae.*
2. *Wound/abdomen.* The commonest organisms involved are *Staph. aureus*, Gram-negative bacilli like *E. coli* and anaerobes.
3. *Urine.* Particularly after catheterization or any urinary tract instrumentation, the commonest organisms are again the Gram-negatives like *E. coli*.
4. *Lines.* Line infection should be considered in any patient with a central line, particularly if it has been in place for over a week.
5. *CNS.* Should be considered after neurosurgery, especially after insertion of ventriculo-peritoneal shunt.
6. *Extremities.* Ischaemic limbs can harbour sepsis, especially with anaerobes

such as *Clostridium welchii*. Orthopaedic implants can get infected.

7. *Other.* For a patient who originally presented with abdominal pain, and particularly if they went on to have a laparotomy which was negative, it is worth considering other weird causes of abdominal pain and fever (e.g. typhoid or malaria). Bacterial endocarditis is a risk in patients with heart valve abnormalities.

Assessment

1. *Temperature.* The level and nature of the fever gives important clues. Because low-grade fever is common postoperatively, investigation and treatment is only necessary if the temperature is 38°C or greater, under normal circumstances. An axillary temperature is unreliable, and tends to be an underestimate. Insist on oral, rectal or tympanic measurements. A swinging pyrexia suggests an abscess.
2. *Relevant history.* This means nature of surgery, recent microbiological history (check recent antibiotics and look for microbiology reports in the notes), and existence of any special problems, that is immuno-suppression, burns, splenectomy.
3. *Other signs of toxaemia.* Tachycardia, tachypnoea, warm peripheries, bounding pulse, rigors, hypotension.
4. *Clues as to focus.* Cough/sputum, chest signs, dysuria or 'mucky-looking urine'. Inflamed-looking pus-y[a] wound, peritonism, meningism, long-standing central line.
5. *Other tests.* When in doubt. For example white cell count, C-reactive protein (a highly sensitive but non-specific indicator of infection or inflammation), chest X-ray.

Specimens

These are the key to good microbiology practice. The type of specimen taken will depend on the suspected focus, if any. There is widespread confusion about which specimens to take and what to do with them.

The single biggest problem is the practice of starting empirical treatment with antibiotics without taking appropriate specimens first. This causes considerable difficulty later on, delays effective treatment and may lead to antibiotic resistance.

Blood cultures. This is the most effective tool when used properly. On the whole we do not take enough.

Significant fevers (i.e. >38°C) can be caused by the presence of tiny numbers of organisms in the peripheral blood. The chance of catching one is about 60–70% with a 10 ml venepuncture. Blood cultures can become contaminated by normal skin flora, and false positive results are common.

However, in some hospitals, blood cultures are expected to be taken with an absurdly convoluted rigmarole that resembles a Russian Orthodox baptism, and takes about an hour. Not surprising, therefore, that harassed house officers decide against taking them altogether. There is no evidence that surgical-style scrubbing up, draping, incantations, etc., have a significant

---

[a] You would not believe the arguments that went on as to how this very useful word should be spelt. I'm still not sure we got it right.

effect on specificity. The technique described below is acceptable, and takes no longer than a set of bloods.

- Place the tourniquet, prepare a wide area of skin. Note if you are using alcohol it is essential to **let it dry** first. Alcohol works by desiccation.
- Wash your hands and put on sterile gloves.
- Take 10 ml of blood, discard the needle. Place 5 ml in each bottle, using a fresh needle each time. You can take blood for other tests at the same time, but it is important to fill the blood cultures first, as other blood bottles are not sterile.
- It is not essential to take two venepunctures, though this will improve chances of a positive result. Don't take the sample from any kind of line, as the results are almost impossible to interpret.

The best time to take a blood culture is at the peak of bacteraemia, which for a patient with 'spiking' fevers, is just *before* the peak of temperature. Blood cultures should be placed in an incubator immediately.

Urine. Generally, a mid-stream urine specimen is useful, sensitive and specific. The finding of significant white cells indicates urinary tract infection, even if no organisms are seen or grown. A catheter specimen is less useful, as white cells may be a normal finding. Urgent microscopy and Gram stain is rarely indicated and samples can be refrigerated overnight.

Sputum. This rarely yields useful results, as sputum is always full of normal flora, and some pathogens may colonize the respiratory tract. Urgent microscopy or Gram staining is never indicated. The only truly significant result is a heavy growth of a known respiratory pathogen. Note that blood cultures are a **much** more productive way to investigate suspected pneumonia.

Cerebrospinal fluid. This is collected by lumbar puncture or from a CSF reservoir in cases of suspected meningitis, which is rare in the perioperative period. It should be sent for microscopy and Gram staining immediately.

Wound swabs. Frank pus yields good results. Optimistically wiping an erythematous area usually only grows skin commensals.

Non-antibiotic treatment

For certain infections, non-antibiotic treatment may be just as important as drugs:

- Chest infection: sputum clearance is the key (see Chapter II.17), which means **good analgesia** and physiotherapy.
- Wound infection: pus needs to be released, which can be done by removing one or more sutures. Deep seated intra-abdominal sepsis (like all abscesses) requires surgical exploration and drainage.
- Urinary tract infection: treatment is more effective if the catheter can be removed. A higher urine output helps, also. Alkalization of the urine, for example with mist. Pot. Cit., helps symptoms of dysuria.
- 'Line infection': an infected CVP line must be removed as part of the management. The tip should be cut off and sent for culture.

Antibiotic treatment

Don't even *read* this unless you have already taken your specimens.

The most straightforward situation is when you have a culture and sensitivity report in front of you. Then appropriate antibiotics can be started straight away. More commonly, however, you have to choose a 'best guess' antibiotic to cover until the culture information is available. For the house surgeon, it can be pruned down to a choice of two scenarios:

1. There is a significant fever (>38°C) in a postoperative patient who has had no recent antibiotic therapy (other than prophylaxis) and has no special problems. Wound, chest or urine are suspected.

    The first choice drug is good ol' **cefuroxime**. This provides useful cover for *Staph. aureus*, *E. coli* and the Gram negatives, and *Strep. pneumoniae*. These organisms are responsible for the majority of perioperative infections. *Note:* a decent dose is required, that is 1.5 g i.v., three times a day.

    If you suspect anaerobes may be responsible (e.g. after gastrointestinal surgery, abdominal wound infections) add **metronidazole** 500 mg, i.v. or p.r.

    If the patient received cefuroxime as perioperative prophylaxis, it is probably a good idea to use something different, for example **augmentin** 1.2 g, three times a day.

2. The situation is complicated by:
    - recent course of antibiotic therapy (other than prophylaxis);
    - immunosuppression or neutropoenia;
    - serious illness, septic shock, burns, multi-organ failure;
    - failure of treatment;
    - known allergy to first-line agents;
    - known resistant organism or contact (e.g. MRSA);
    - unusual focus of infection (e.g. brain abscess), or suspected weird diagnosis (e.g. typhoid).

In this case, the advice is even simpler: speak to the microbiologist. He or she can guide you with further investigations as well as therapy. Microbiologists are famously happy to give advice and would much prefer to be involved early, in order to avoid problems with diagnosis or resistant organisms later.

Chapter II.20

HYPOTHERMIA

Chapter II.20

HYPOTHERMIA

KEY POINTS

Hypothermia is a common, serious and often insidious occurrence amongst surgical patients, which contributes significantly to perioperative morbidity.

Think of it in any unwell postoperative patient. Do not accept axillary temperature measurements.

Treat it with oxygen, warm blankets, warm intravenous fluids and a woolly hat. The fluid requirement will be greater than expected during rewarming.

Definitions

- Mild: 35–37°C.
- Moderate: 32–35°C.
- Severe: <32°C.

Causes

Surgical patients, especially elderly trauma victims, are occasionally admitted from the community with a low core temperature, but most frequently hypothermia occurs as a consequence of anaesthesia and surgery.

During anaesthesia, basal metabolic rate is considerably reduced, limiting heat production. The hypothalamic temperature regulation mechanisms are altered, and many of the normal responses to hypothermia (shivering, piloerection, cutaneous vasoconstriction) are inhibited.

When body cavities are opened, there is a considerable evaporative heat loss, and often large areas of skin are exposed. The use of unwarmed, i.v. fluid (especially blood), and ventilation with unhumidified gas all further contribute to heat loss.

Patients at particular risk are:

- Those at the extremes of age. Babies because of their higher surface area/ weight ratio, and the elderly because of reduced ability to generate heat.
- Thoracic or abdominal surgery.
- Prolonged surgery.
- Emergency surgery, especially trauma.
- After massive blood transfusion.
- Those with some medical conditions (e.g. hypothyroidism and malnutrition).

Effects

Cardiovascular. In mild or moderate hypothermia, the predominant effect is an increase in myocardial oxygen demand, as a result of vasoconstriction and shivering. Progressive cooling, however, leads to a gradual drop in pulse, blood pressure and cardiac output. Severe hypothermia causes dysrhythmias, and spontaneous ventricular fibrillation occurs at temperatures of <28°C. Blood viscosity increases.

Respiratory. In mild or moderate hypothermia, shivering dramatically increases overall oxygen consumption, and can lead to severe hypoxaemia. (Any shivering patient should be given oxygen.) With lower temperatures, there is progressive depression of ventilation, but the fall in oxygen delivery is matched by the drop in metabolic rate. The oxyhaemoglobin dissociation curve is shifted to the left, which reduces the availability of oxygen to the tissues.

Central nervous system. There is a progressive depression of consciousness with severe hypothermia. The pupils may become fixed and dilated below 28°C.

Other. Clotting function is reduced. Renal and hepatic function are progressively reduced, which reduces the elimination of most drugs. Serum potassium rises, pH falls, and the metabolism of lactate and citrate is reduced. Glucose utilization is reduced, which may lead to hyperglycaemia.

Technical problems. Blood pressure measurement is difficult. Automatic blood pressure devices misread in shivering patients. Pulse oximeters may fail or give inaccurate readings due to poor peripheral perfusion. Venepuncture and venflon siting are difficult.

Measurement of body temperature

It is unlikely that a seriously hypothermic patient will not be recognized as such. However, more commonly you will be called to see a postoperative patient who is non-specifically unwell, and an important part of improving the overall condition is to recognize and treat any element of hypothermia.

A low body temperature is harder to demonstrate than a fever. **Never** accept an axillary temperature measurement as a valid reflection of core temperature. Axillary temperatures are often taken on sick patients who can't co-operate with an oral measurement. This practice should be strongly discouraged.

The following provide useful measurement of core temperature:
- Oral thermometer in an alert and co-operative patient.
- Rectal thermometer, less pleasant but reliable.
- Infrared tympanic membrane thermometer. This device is accurate, quick, reliable, and can be used on any patient.
- Nasopharyngeal or oesophageal temperature probes. Only really of use in the unconscious, ventilated patient, but the results are reliable.

Management

The hypothermic patient should be given oxygen.

Passive rewarming. This is suitable for most cases of postoperative hypothermia. The aim is to minimize heat loss, and avoid any iatrogenic cooling. Place the patient in a warm room (25–30°C), cover completely. Aluminium 'space blankets' are often used, though woollen ones are just as good. Remember to cover the body's most effective radiator – the scalp. The requirement for i.v. fluid will be greater than expected, and all fluids should be warmed to 37°C. Many people fail to understand that by giving a hypothermic patient fluids at room temperature (20°C), you are *cooling them down*.

Active surface rewarming. This may be necessary for young patients with moderate hypothermia, or for those who have not responded to passive rewarming. It involves use of electric blankets, heated mattresses, or even warm baths. Most hospitals now have one or two 'Bair Huggers®' in recovery or ITU. These devices work by blowing warm air through a special blanket, and are extremely effective.

Active rewarming of extremities can cause abrupt vasodilation and hypotension, for which the treatment is fluid challenge. Reperfusion of cold extremities can actually lead to a drop in core temperature ('after drop'), and a worsening of acidosis. This phenomenon can also be observed after release of an arterial tourniquet during limb surgery. Active heating of poorly perfused areas can also lead to skin burns.

Active core rewarming. Theoretically, a method which warms the core before the extremities ensures that the vital organs recover before extra demands are made of them. The only practical method of achieving this, however, is with cardiopulmonary bypass, or some other extracorporeal circulation. It is reserved for use in severe hypothermia associated with cardiac arrest.

Chapter II.21

CENTRAL NERVOUS SYSTEM COMPLICATIONS

Chapter II.21

CENTRAL NERVOUS SYSTEM COMPLICATIONS

KEY POINTS

Delirium is always due to an systemic organic disorder until proven otherwise.

Actively seek an underlying cause of delirium, do not just treat the symptoms.

Coma is never a normal finding, nor is it safe to attribute it to anaesthesia.

Convulsions: all that fits is not epilepsy.

Introduction

The division of a whole organism into organ systems is convenient when classifying problems, but is somewhat artificial. Thus the commonest postoperative 'central nervous system' complications are actually CNS manifestations of dysfunction in other systems. Most causes of CNS symptoms are reversible, which makes it all the more important to diagnose the true cause and not just to treat the symptoms blindly.

This chapter will deal with delirium, sleep problems, coma, convulsions and extra-pyramidal symptoms.

"Doctor, Mrs Smith is very confused"

First, a word on definitions. *Delirium* is a term used to describe a syndrome of acute, fluctuating disturbance of attention, memory, sleep, orientation, perception and psychomotor function. It has replaced terms like 'acute confusion', 'organic brain disease' and 'gone crazy'. Delirium usually occurs in the first few days postop, often after a lucid interval. It is typically worst at night, when you are most likely to get a call about it. Not all patients will be agitated. Some will be withdrawn, causing difficulty in recognizing the problem.

Dementia differs from delirium in having a gradual onset and in being largely irreversible. It also shows as a global cerebral impairment.

Depression may co-exist with or mimic either delirium or dementia. Many of the symptoms overlap (sleep disturbance, withdrawal, inattentiveness, agitation) and confuse the diagnosis.

"Thanks, Doc, but Mrs Smith is still confused"

To get the correct answer you will need to follow a set of diagnostic steps:

Is Mrs Smith really confused?

Not everyone with strange ideas is delirious. Not everyone who fails to communicate is depressed (they might be deaf or be on the other side of a language or culture barrier). Check it out for yourself with a set of simple tests of memory and orientation: ask your patient's age, the time, the date, the name of the hospital and of the reigning monarch. Ask the year of a *major* historical event (one relevant to the patient's background). Ask them to identify staff members by their uniforms (e.g. doctor, nurse), to remember an address and repeat it later, and to count backwards from 20.

Is this delirium or dementia?

This shouldn't be too difficult if you took a decent history on admission. Delirium is an acute syndrome; dementia is chronic. The family can be very useful in giving a comparison between the present and the preop states, and in spilling the beans about alcohol or drug intake. Remember that dementia may appear to worsen in unfamiliar surroundings and that demented people can also suffer delirium.

OK, it's delirium. Why?

Dysfunction in almost any system can manifest as delirium; possible causes are:

- **Metabolic:** hypoglycaemia, hyperglycaemia, dehydration, hyponatraemia, uraemia, acidosis, hypophosphataemia, hypercalcaemia, hypocalcaemia, hypothyroidism, hyperthyroidism, liver failure, porphyria.
- **Respiratory:** hypoxia, infection, pulmonary embolus, fat embolus.
- **Infections:** respiratory, urinary, wounds, intra-abdominal.
- **Cardiac:** myocardial infarct, heart failure, hypotension.
- **Neurological:** raised intracranial pressure, brain contusion, reduced perfusion, post-ictal state, CVA/TIA, post-cardiac bypass, infection, sensory/sleep deprivation.
- **Excretory:** urinary retention, constipation.
- **Drugs:** iatrogenic (see below), withdrawal (alcohol, benzodiazepines, opioids).

To sort out the cause you will need to perform a thorough physical examination of all the systems involved above. Be particularly suspicious of hypoxia, infections, dehydration and urinary retention as one of these is frequently the culprit. Your next step is a review of the drug chart. Consider drug withdrawal as well as iatrogenic delirium. Drugs which most commonly cause delirium include:

- **Analgesics:** opioids (especially pethidine).
- **Local anaesthetics:** in overdose.
- **Psychotropics:** benzodiazepines, tricyclics, haloperidol.
- **Anti-emetics:** prochlorperazine, metoclopramide, droperidol.
- **Anticholinergics:** atropine, hyoscine.
- **Steroids.**

Investigations may be the only way to determine the cause of delirium in some cases, or may confirm clinical findings. In all cases, hypoxia, electrolyte imbalance, myocardial ischaemia and infection need to be actively excluded.

- **FBC:** anaemia (decreased oxygen carriage, liver disease, alcohol), white cell count.
- **U&Es:** dehydration and electrolyte imbalance.
- **Glucose:** hypoglycaemia, hyperglycaemia.
- **Urinalysis:** both for microbiology and for chemistry.
- **Gases:** ± oximetry for hypoxia or acidosis.
- **ECG :** ± enzymes for ischaemia, infarct or dysrhythmia.
- **Radiology:** chest X-ray ultrasounds, CT scans, V/Q scans.
- **Biochemistry:** thyroid function, LFT, drug screening, porphyrins.

Principles of treating delirium

Treatment takes two forms: dealing with the cause of the delirium appropriately (see chapters on electrolytes, fluids, metabolism, etc.), and giving supportive care to prevent deterioration or injury as long as the patient remains delirious.

Nursing care
Nurses have a lot to offer in minimizing the risk of injury (e.g. cot bumpers, tricks to protect i.v. access and to maintain oxygen therapy) and also may have experience in techniques to minimize disorientation. Less experienced nurses may be inclined to rely too much on sedation and should be politely resisted until you are sure that it is indicated. Restraints are very rarely a good idea; they worsen the agitation and increase the risks of injury.

Rehydration
Dehydration causes delirium and delirium causes dehydration. Good fluid and electrolyte control is essential and is likely to need secure i.v. access, repeated investigations and measurement of urine output. This can be awkward with an unco-operative patient.

Oxygen
Hypoxia is common, especially at night (see Chapter II.17). All patients who have had major surgery should receive oxygen at night. All delirious patients should have at least a trial of oxygen, along with serial gases or oximetry, to find if they are helped by it. Persistent hypoxia with delirium despite oxygen is likely to mean a transfer to ITU.

Nutrition and vitamins
Adequate calorie and protein intake needs to be continued, often by the nasogastric route; the help of a dietician is invaluable. **Vitamin B$_{12}$** may be indicated if there is good evidence of alcoholism or chronic deficiency.

Sedatives
Sedation should be a last resort, not an automatic reaction to delirium. Note that most sedatives can cause delirium and that many are respiratory depressants. When sedation is essential it is best given in regular small doses. Benzodiazepines are respiratory depressants, long-acting and disturb normal cognitive function; unless they are specifically indicated they should be

avoided. **Haloperidol** is a good choice and can be given orally in doses of 0.5–2.0 mg 6-hourly. **Thioridazine** is an alternative in doses of 5–10 mg 8-hourly. This dose can be increased to a maximum of 30 mg 8-hourly, but be careful not to cause oversedation in the elderly.

Withdrawal

Withdrawal from alcohol, opioids or from benzodiazepines is a 'special case' in causation of delirium and deserves a further mention.

Alcohol
Alcohol withdrawal leads to a range of problems and severe cases are life-threatening. Alcoholic tremor is like a bad hangover, with shaking, headache, foul mood and bad breath; it just requires fluids, paracetamol, and maybe thiamine. Alcoholic hallucinosis usually presents as auditory hallucinations in someone who is otherwise unaffected. **Haloperidol** is a useful symptomatic treatment.

Often alcohol withdrawals result in convulsions. These are generalized and often resistant to anticonvulsants. The treatment of choice is a benzodiazepine (e.g. **diazepam** 10–20 mg i.v. *slowly*). Remember that, in an emergency, diazepam can be given rectally (10–20 mg) but is of limited value intramuscularly. You are now going to need expert help from psychiatry and/ or ITU.

Most dreaded of all is delirium tremens (the DTs). This still carries a mortality of 2%. It presents as full-blown delirium, with or without fitting, 3–5 days after the last drink. It is a diagnosis of exclusion. **Benzodiazepines** are specifically indicated as above. You will need expert help.

Benzodiazepine withdrawal
These drugs are in very common use among the general public, and dependence on them is rife, even though patients and family may be unaware of it. The simplest strategy is to continue whichever agent is used at home during the hospital stay and to advise a discussion with the GP on discharge. The withdrawal syndrome is very unpleasant; anxiety, sweating, restlessness, nightmares and fever are common. Convulsions, hallucinations and delirium may occur. Weaning is *inappropriate* in the perioperative period and is best done very gradually, by an expert, after recovery from surgery.

Opioid withdrawal
'Cold turkey' is said to feel like a bad case of 'flu. Anxiety, fatigue, aching, hypertension, tachycardia, rhinorrhoea and diarrhoea are common. Any opioid can be used to prevent withdrawal symptoms (see Chapter II.4) and maintain analgesia. Refer the patient for weaning at a later date; do not attempt to restrict opioids in the postoperative period. What you should be aiming for is the prevention of withdrawal syndromes, not a treatment of the addiction.

"Doctor, Mrs Smith can't sleep"

To which the obvious answer is: "Neither can I". Various things make sleeping in hospital difficult. The beds are hard; the wards are noisy and lack privacy. Pain, anxiety and depression often afflict the surgical patient. Any of the causes of delirium may also disturb sleep (see above). Many patients just have unrealistic expectations; 8 h of dreamless oblivion are impossible on a surgical ward. Withdrawal from alcohol, benzodiazepines or other psychotropic drugs is very common. Many drugs cause restlessness through a central excitation; caffeine is an obvious example. Aminophylline, amphetamines, doxapram, inotropes and other β-agonists such as salbutamol can also cause arousal.

Having checked that the cause of the insomnia is not pain, delirium or depression you will need to choose a hypnotic agent. Although many drugs are sedative the useful night sedatives are few.

Benzodiazepines

As well as their hypnotic and anxiolytic actions, these have the advantage of preventing alcohol withdrawal syndromes. It is essential to pick a short-acting agent to avoid daytime sedation. If a patient is receiving a long-acting benzodiazepine (e.g. diazepam) for another reason, you should make sure that the dose is given at night; otherwise stick with short-acting agents. A suitable choice is *temazepam* (10–20 mg). Problems include respiratory depression and addiction. All patients must be warned that the hypnotics are extremely habit-forming and should be used infrequently, irregularly and only in the short term. Reduce the dose in the elderly, and avoid benzodiazepines altogether when respiratory function is critical.

Chloral, triclofos and chlormethiazole

Chloral hydrate and its derivative *triclofos* have traditionally been used for the elderly and for children, but they have no real advantage over the benzodiazepines. They are addictive and contraindicated by severe respiratory disease. *Chlormethiazole* is less habit-forming than the benzodiazepines and has a short duration, which makes it a useful alternative for the elderly. Severe reactions may occur if it is taken with alcohol.

Other sedative drugs

Tricyclic antidepressants have sedative properties and improve sleep in depressed patients, but they are not indicated for simple insomnia. Be sure to prescribe them as an 8 p.m. dose to utilize the sedation and avoid daytime drowsiness. *Antihistamines* should also be given at night for the same reasons. *Opioid analgesics* are powerful respiratory depressants and should be used as sedatives only in high-dependency areas such as ITU. *Thioridazine* in low doses has useful sedative action although this is not its primary indication. It is reasonable to allow small amounts of *alcohol* to those who are used to an evening drink.

"Doctor, Mrs Smith won't wake up"

The causes of a depressed level of consciousness, like those of delirium, are many and the patient should be approached in the same way, with a thorough examination and relevant investigations. The primary problem may be metabolic, neurological, cardiovascular, infective or drug intoxication (as listed above). Knowing the patient's history gives invaluable clues; you might suspect raised intracranial pressure as a cause following trauma, or electrolyte imbalance after urological surgery. Coma is never a normal finding, *nor is it safe to attribute it to anaesthesia.* Anaesthetic drugs are very short acting and the patients are not discharged from recovery until their effects have worn off.

When there is good reason to suspect drug-induced coma (e.g. the clinical picture of narcotism), a therapeutic trial of a specific antagonist is reasonable. Intravenous *naloxone* (0.1–0.2 mg) reverses opioid sedation, but also the analgesia. Naloxone has a short duration of action and repeated doses or an infusion may be needed. *Flumazenil* (200 mcg i.v.) reverses the effects of benzodiazepines. It can precipitate a withdrawal syndrome in chronic benzodiazepine users and, like naloxone, has a very short duration of action.

Any comatose patient is at risk of respiratory arrest, airway obstruction, aspiration and dehydration. If coma persists, you should think hard about referring to ITU. This has the added advantage of letting you get back to bed.

"Doctor, Mrs Smith won't stop twitching"

Convulsions
All that fits is not epilepsy. Causes of convulsions are:
- **Neurological:** brain contusion, infections, raised intracranial pressure, epilepsy, CVA.
- **Drugs:** many agents in overdose, for example lithium, tricyclics, aminophylline, NSAIDs, anti-emetics, local anaesthetics.
- **Withdrawal:** commonly alcohol.
- **Metabolic:** hyponatraemia, hypoglycaemia, hypercalcaemia, hypomagnesaemia.
- **Respiratory:** hypoxia, alkalosis.
- **Infection:** febrile convulsions in children.
- **Pregnancy:** eclampsia.

Emergency treatment includes maintenance of a clear airway, supplemental oxygen and prevention of injury. The emergency drug of choice is *diazepam* (10–20 mg i.v. slowly or 10–20 mg p.r.). This can be followed by *phenytoin* (15 mg/kg i.v. very slowly). Continued fitting may require *paraldehyde*, *chlormethiazole* or even general anaesthesia. The cause of the fit must be vigorously pursued with clinical and laboratory tests. **Don't forget a pregnancy test in young women.**

Extrapyramidal problems

Pre-existing Parkinsonism may worsen during a surgical admission due to difficulty in administering the drugs. Extrapyramidal symptoms such as rigidity, tremor, dystonia, akathisia, tardive dyskinesia and oculogyric crisis may be precipitated by many drugs used perioperatively; notably anti-emetics (droperidol, metoclopramide, prochlorperazine), and antipsychotics (chlorpromazine, haloperidol). These should be used with caution in the elderly and avoided whenever possible in Parkinsonian patients. Antimuscarinics such as *procyclidine* (5–10 mg i.m.) are used to treat symptoms of drug-induced Parkinsonism.

Chapter II.22

MISCELLANEOUS POSTOPERATIVE PROBLEMS

MISCELLANEOUS POSTOPERATIVE PROBLEMS

Thyroidectomy problems

Apart from the complications you can expect from any operation (sepsis, bleeding, anaesthetic disasters), thyroidectomy can cause special problems that are divided into two groups.

Airway obstruction. This may be due to:
* Postoperative haematoma. This may be dramatic. The management is to remove the skin closure clips and evacuate the clot at the bedside.
* Laryngeal oedema. This sometimes occurs on the 2nd or 3rd day and is gradual in onset. Severe stridor may necessitate tracheostomy.
* Recurrent laryngeal nerve injury. This is not uncommon, but is usually unilateral and often transient. Complete, bilateral damage may result in adducted cords and airway obstruction. Patients usually have cord function assessed by an ENT surgeon before thyroidectomy.
* Tracheomalacia. A very large long-standing goitre may erode the tracheal cartilages, and when the gland is removed, the trachea collapses on inspiration. Not funny.

Hormonal problems.
* Thyroid crisis. This is now rare, as a toxic gland is rarely operated upon. Clinical features include fever, tachycardia, dysrhythmias, abdominal pain and diarrhoea. Treatment is with β-blockers, iodide and steroids. Help from an endocrinologist and intensive care should be sought. The mortality is extremely high.
* Hypoparathyroidism. If all four parathyroid glands are removed, hypocalcaemia will result. It is worth checking serum calcium post-operatively. Severe hypocalcaemia causes tetany. Treatment initially is with 20 ml of 10% calcium gluconate given slowly i.v.

TUR syndrome

This is an important condition that sometimes complicates transurethral resection of the prostate. It occurs as a result of absorption of large quantities of the 1.5% glycine irrigating solution through open venous sinuses. It has an incidence of up to 15% of prostatectomies, and is not uncommonly fatal. The clinical effects are mainly due to haemodilution and hyponatraemia.

Patients in whom resection was prolonged (>1 h) or performed by junior surgeons, patients with a large gland and those with pre-existing hyponatraemia are particularly susceptible. The syndrome has also been described after percutaneous ultrasonic lithotripsy and transcervical resection of endometrium (TCRE). It may present at any time within the first 12 h after surgery.

In a conscious patient, the first signs are restlessness, headache, confusion. Initial cardiovascular signs are a widening of pulse pressure and an increase in systolic pressure. This is followed by hypotension, bradycardia, dysrhythmias and, in severe cases, cardiac arrest. If severe, or untreated, the patient may develop cerebral oedema with convulsions or coma, and pulmonary oedema.

The diagnosis can be confirmed by measurement of plasma sodium. Problems are likely when sodium is <120 mmol/l, but any significant drop should be taken seriously. Blood should be sent for plasma osmolality, which is another guide to severity. Haemoglobin and haematocrit are usually depressed by haemodilution. Fluid management is difficult after TURP, as bleeding certainly occurs, and some patients will be hypovolaemic. Accurate records of intraoperative blood loss are very difficult to obtain.

Management is unfortunately controversial. There are three main therapeutic options:

1. Loop diuretics (e.g. frusemide 40 mg i.v.), given that the majority of patients are overloaded, and the most serious complications (e.g. cerebral oedema) are a consequence of this. However, frusemide causes diuresis by removal of sodium, which is a curious way to treat hyponatraemia.
2. Do nothing. This is based on the knowledge that many patients with severe hyponatraemia (e.g. as low as 104 mmol/l) may be asymptomatic and spontaneously correct the problem, and on the undisputed fact that rapid correction of hyponatraemia is dangerous.
3. Active treatment with saline, either 0.9% ('normal') or, more controversially, 1.8% ('hypertonic'). The big danger here is further volume loading to a patient who may already be overloaded. It has been recommended that the sodium level should not rise more than 2 mmol/l/h.

Clearly, it is not possible to give dogmatic advice, and each case should be treated individually. The biggest disasters, however, occur when no-one even suspects the diagnosis, so spotting the disorder is most of the battle. We recommend:

- For a stable patient with mild hyponatraemia, it is justifiable to do nothing specific. They should receive only the usual maintenance fluid (2000 ml/24 h) but 5% dextrose and dextrose–saline should be avoided. Hesitate to treat a low haemoglobin with blood transfusion unless you are sure that heavy blood loss took place. Regular (e.g. 6-hourly) U&E measurements should be made.
- For patients with clinical evidence such as cardiovascular instability or fits, the patient should be managed on ITU. The difficulties over clinical assessment of volume status make invasive monitoring with CVP, or even Swan–Ganz catheters, justified. Inotropes or calcium may be indicated, and coagulation studies should be performed, as DIC is a recognized complication.

Eye problems

The eye is vulnerable to a wide range of insults during anaesthesia.

Corneal abrasion

This is perhaps the commonest problem. The eye is sore and red, perhaps with a gritty feeling. The diagnosis is readily confirmed by placing a drop of 0.5% amethocaine, followed by fluorescein, in the affected eye. The abrasion will take up the stain. Treatment consists of an eye pad and bandage, and chloramphenicol ointment.

Acute (closed angle) glaucoma
In susceptible patients this presents with severe pain in and around the eye, nausea and vomiting. The cornea may be cloudy and the pupil dilated. This is as close as you get to a true ophthalmological emergency, so get an eye doctor. Emergency treatment is with diuretics such as acetazolamide 500 mg, or 10% mannitol.

Acute blindness
This is rare, and often transient. It may occur due to retinal infarction from prolonged pressure on the eye, from basilar artery spasm, acute multiple sclerosis, or even TUR syndrome. Although there is often no specific treatment, advice from an ophthalmologist should be urgently sought, if only for medico-legal reasons.

Post-intubation problems

Problems caused by intubation may present postoperatively. Sore throat is common (and can occur in patients who weren't intubated), but requires only symptomatic treatment (e.g. Difflam gargle or lozenges). Common injuries include damage to teeth, lips and pharynx. Teeth need to be found, and early in-patient dental treatment offered where possible. Tears in the pharyngeal mucosa can lead to extensive surgical emphysema or retropharyngeal abscess. Damage to the vocal cords may lead to transient hoarseness. Arytenoid dislocation presents with hoarseness and acute pain on swallowing. Early referral to an ENT surgeon is indicated. The recurrent laryngeal nerve may be damaged.

Musculoskeletal problems

Swollen joint(s)
For a single joint, especially in the foot, the most likely cause postoperatively is **gout**. Measure uric acid, and involve a rheumatologist if in doubt. Treatment is with strong NSAIDs (e.g. indomethacin 50 mg t.i.d). The other cause of swollen joints to remember is **septic arthritis**. Here, there will be signs of infection. Treatment is with immobilization, antibiotics and joint aspiration.

Nerve injuries
These can occur as a result of poor positioning, injection of substances into the nerve, or use of tourniquets. Injury can affect the brachial plexus, radial, median or ulnar nerves, the lateral popliteal nerve (leading to footdrop) or sciatic nerve, among others. Occasionally, the supraorbital nerve is damaged, which leads to photophobia, numbness on the forehead and pain in the eye. Full documentation should be made immediately a nerve injury is suspected. Recovery is usual, but may take months.

Anaphylactoid reactions

This is a general term for dramatic, generalized, life-threatening allergic responses, which occur most commonly to i.v. drugs or insect stings. There are two basic types of reaction:

1. Type I hypersensitivity reaction, or true anaphylaxis. In this type, prior exposure to the drug is required. On the first exposure, lymphocytes produce specific IgE antibodies, which attach to the membranes of mast cells and basophils. A second exposure leads to degranulation of mast cells on a massive scale, leading to the clinical effect.
2. Complement-mediated reactions. Here, exposure leads to activation of the complement cascade, with production of the anaphylotoxins C3a and C5a, which cause mast cell degranulation. The important difference is that **prior exposure is not necessary**. Complement-mediated reactions are at least as common as IgE-mediated ones.

Presentation
1. *Skin.* A characteristic urticarial rash or flushing usually appears rapidly.
2. *Cardiovascular system.* The effects vary from hypotension to total cardiovascular collapse. Hypotension is the result of release of histamine and other vasoactive peptides, which cause widespread capillary vasodilation and increased capillary permeability. Leakage of fluid may cause significant extracellular fluid loss. Dysrhythmias may occur, most commonly supraventricular tachycardia.
3. *Bronchospasm*, may be life-threatening.
4. *Glottic oedema*, occasionally occurs, threatening the airway.
5. *Gastrointestinal.* Immediately after recovery, the patient may complain of abdominal pain, diarrhoea, nausea and vomiting.
6. *Miscellaneous.* Other effects include conduction defects, coagulation disorders and leukopoenia.

Management
Immediate:
1. Discontinue administration of suspected drugs, give oxygen and maintain the airway.
2. Call a cardiac arrest. This is the easiest and quickest way to get everything you need to manage the patient, that is adrenaline, monitoring, pairs of hands, and senior assistance.
3. Give adrenaline. This is the drug of choice for all but the mildest of reactions, and it opposes all the pathological effects of anaphylaxis. There is good evidence that the earlier the adrenaline is given, the better the outcome. For in-hospital anaphylaxis, and where there is venous access, adrenaline should be given i.v., **not** i.m., subcutaneously or anywhere else. The initial i.v. dose should be 0.1 mg, which is 1 ml of 1 in 10 000, given in increments of 0.1 mg. (The preloaded Minijet syringes contain 1 in 10 000.) An ECG monitor should be applied as soon as possible. Adrenaline has a short action, and repeated doses may be necessary.
4. Give i.v. fluid, for example 1–2 litres of saline stat. Decent venous access is required (14- or 16-gauge). Colloid solutions may be preferable if available.
5. Glottic oedema may require intubation or cricothyroidotomy.

Second-line management:

1. Antihistamines. These are normally given, but only partially reverse the effects, as histamine is not the only mediator involved. The agent of choice is chlorpheniramine (Piriton) 10–20 mg slowly i.v. Do not fumble around looking for Piriton when the patient is dying.

2. Aminophylline may be required for persistent bronchospasm, particularly in the absence of hypotension; 5 mg/kg can be given over 20 min.

3. Steroids. These have no place in immediate management, as they take several hours to work. They may be given if the reaction persists, for example hydrocortisone 200 mg i.v.

4. Investigations. It may be desirable to take blood samples to confirm the diagnosis, and identify the agent responsible. This is particularly important when multiple drugs have been given in quick succession (e.g. after induction of anaesthesia). Some hospitals perform the required tests on site, so contact your pathology or immunology department for further advice. Two EDTA (pink top) blood samples should be taken immediately after the reaction, and again at 3, 6, 12 and 24 h. It is very useful to have a pre-event sample, so try to get hold of any recent full blood count samples from the haematology lab. Skin testing may be appropriate, but only if recommended and carried out by an expert in the investigation of drug allergies.

5. Where a drug is implicated with reasonable certainty, the patient should be informed. Suggest a Medic Alert bracelet. Full documentation should be made in (and on the cover of) the notes. Inform the patient's general practitioner.

Tracheostomy

Patients may return to the surgical ward with either permanent or temporary tracheostomies. The former is performed as part of radical neck surgery such as laryngectomy, and the latter following brain, face or neck injury or prolonged ventilation. Tracheostomy causes many difficulties.

With most types of tube there is no airflow through the larynx, so the patient cannot speak. Make sure writing materials and a bell are available. Later in the recovery 'fenestrated' tubes that allow speech can be used.

Because a build-up and sudden release of pressure within the airway cannot be achieved with an open tracheostomy tube, a normal cough is not possible. Regular suctioning and physiotherapy are needed to prevent sputum retention.

Dysphagia is common due to the bulk of the cuff and to poorly co-ordinated swallowing. This can be partly relieved by temporarily deflating the cuff. As this may leave the airway unprotected from soiling, it is important to assess swallowing before allowing solids. We use a highly coloured liquid (e.g. Ribena), ask the patient to swallow, observe for coughing, and then examine the tracheal aspirate for colouration.

The presence of a foreign body in the airway is irritating and causes secretions. These form hard crusts if allowed to collect and can obstruct the tube. Humidification and regular suctioning are effective in prevention.

Pressure necrosis of the trachea is caused by a poorly positioned tube or an overinflated cuff. This can result in stenosis or oedema which make extubation impossible. Erosion into the front of the neck can lead to fatal haemorrhage. Therefore, check the cuff pressure regularly and do not let it exceed 20 cmH$_2$O.

Fixing the tube in place is most important in the early stages. Sutures are the best method. Ribbons may become loose as neck swelling decreases or as position changes.

Changing the tube can be hazardous. The tissue planes can shift on removing the old tube so that the track disappears. A common mistake is to try to place the new tube too far anteriorly, which results in cannulation of the anterior mediastinum and no useful airway. To intubate the trachea you need to direct the tube first posteriorly until it reaches the back wall of the trachea (a depth of 3–4 cm), and then turn it inferiorly. The first few times you try it you should get supervision from an ENT surgeon or an anaesthetist. If you are faced with an obstructed tracheostomy put out a crash call. Check the tube for obvious blockage, then try to pass a suction catheter through it. A narrow lumen will keep the patient alive until help arrives. Only as a last resort should you attempt a tube change yourself.

All cases with fresh tracheostomies must be managed with the help of expert nurses. Ask either the ENT ward or ITU for advice.

Chapter II.23

THROMBOSIS

Chapter II.23

THROMBOSIS

KEY POINTS

Deep vein thromboses and pulmonary emboli kill people, and are common in the perioperative period.

As the houseman, it will fall to you to make sure that no high-risk patients escape adequate prophylaxis.

Subcutaneous heparin, TED stockings, dextran, inflatable bootees and epidural analgesia all reduce the incidence of DVT.

Background

Thromboembolic complications are a common consequence of anaesthesia and surgery, occurring in up to 25% of all surgical procedures. This high incidence is the result both of abnormal blood flow, from immobility or operative positioning, and an increase in coagulability of blood as a result of raised fibrinogen, decreased fibrinolysis and increased platelet adhesiveness.

DVT causes morbidity and increased hospital stay and may lead to pulmonary embolus, which may in turn be fatal. Seven percent of all postoperative deaths are the result of pulmonary embolus.

It often falls to the houseman to identify and provide protection for those at greatest risk. Virchow's triad is all very well, but it will not necessarily remind you of all the highest-risk groups.

High-risk groups

1. *Orthopaedic surgery* carries an incidence of 40–75%. The more prolonged the surgery, the greater the risk. Major joint surgery is the most risky.
2. *Gynaecological surgery* particularly in the over-40s.
3. *Cardiac failure.*
4. *Malignancy.*
5. *Obesity.*
6. *The elderly, strokes and generalized immobility.*
7. *Pregnancy or oestrogen therapy* doubles the risk of DVT. To minimize risk in those on the oral contraceptive pill, the drug should be withdrawn at least **6 weeks** before surgery. A shorter abstinence actually increases the risk, as there is a transient *increase* in coagulability after withdrawal of exogenous oestrogen. The problem with stopping the pill is the risk of pregnancy. This issue should be discussed with your consultant, but there is little evidence to support stopping the pill for healthy young women undergoing minor surgery. It is reasonable to advise withdrawal (of the

medication, I mean) where a second risk factor exists.

Hormone-replacement therapy and progesterone-only contraceptives do not increase the risk of DVT.

8. *Peripheral vascular disease and varicose veins.*
9. *Those with a history of DVT or PE.*
10. *Weird things:* antithrombin III deficiency, lupus anticoagulant, protein C deficiency, protein S deficiency. All as rare as rocking-horse whatnots.

Prevention

General measures to reduce the risk in susceptible individuals should be attempted, for example losing weight, adequately treating heart failure or sepsis, withholding oestrogen therapy. All patients should be encouraged to mobilize early, or at least to perform leg exercises whilst in bed. Adequate pain control promotes early mobilization.

Specific measures include:

- Low-dose unfractionated heparin, for example Minihep, 5000 units twice daily, for 5 days. This more than halves the incidence of DVT, and reduces the mortality from PE. It has been estimated that six deaths per 1000 patients undergoing major surgery could be prevented with Minihep.

  Use of heparin is not without problems; wound haematomas are more common, for example, but overall mortality from haemorrhage is not increased. Thrombocytopoenia occurs in 0.3% of patients on low-dose heparin.

- Low molecular weight heparins, for example dalteparin (Fragmin). These agents work in a slightly different way, and have a number of advantages over unfractionated heparin. They can often be given on a once-daily basis, and have been shown to be even more effective at preventing DVT than unfractionated heparin, without any increase in haemorrhagic complications. Although the effects on the incidence of PE are not yet known conclusively, it is likely that low molecular weight heparins will become the agents of choice for prophylaxis.

- Graduated compression ('TED') stockings, if correctly fitted and if worn from before surgery to full mobilization, also reduce the incidence of DVT though an effect on the rate of PE has not been demonstrated. There is some evidence that the benefits of stockings and heparin are additive.

- Intermittent pneumatic compression boots also reduce the incidence. Curiously, they also work when placed on the arm, which suggests an action beyond the simple 'pumping' effect.

- Dextran 40 and 70 both reduce DVT and PE by an antiplatelet effect. Disadvantages with this are the need for i.v. access, allergic reactions, increased bleeding and interference with cross-matching.

- Epidural or spinal anaesthesia, by improving flow and enhancing fibrinolysis.

- Warfarin is effective, but the risk of haemorrhagic complications is greater, and continuous laboratory monitoring is required. It is sometimes used in patients who are a long-term risk (e.g. spinal injury patients).

For most patients, the combination of subcutaneous heparin and TED stockings is highly effective.

Diagnosis and management of thromboembolic complications

DVT can occur in any vein of the leg, but are most common in calf veins. The clinical features are:

1. *None at all.* DVT is commonly asymptomatic.
2. *Pain in the calf*, often presenting with redness, swelling and engorged superficial veins. The affected calf is often warmer and there may be ankle oedema. Homan's sign (pain in the calf on dorsiflexion of the foot) is usually positive, but this is not diagnostic, and is positive with other lesions in the calf.
3. *Groin pain*, in the case of iliofemoral thrombosis, which can be severe and associated with ankle oedema.
4. *Cyanotic discoloration*, of the affected limb may occur with complete occlusion of a large vein.

Pulmonary embolus may occur after any DVT but is rare where the thrombus is confined to the calf. However, calf DVTs may extend proximally without obvious clinical signs.

The investigation of choice is venography and, as it is usually not available immediately the diagnosis is made, treatment with heparin is usually started wherever a suspicion exists. If the diagnosis is confirmed, treatment with anticoagulants is normally continued for 3 months.

The diagnosis and management of pulmonary embolus is covered in Chapter II.17.

Chapter II.24

TRICKS WITH DRIPS

Chapter II.24

TRICKS WITH DRIPS

KEY POINTS

Use local anaesthetic, gloves and a decent tourniquet.
Know when to give up.
Know who to ask when you do.

Introduction

Intravenous cannulae are probably the most frequent of the little tortures that we inflict on the general public in the name of health care. They cause considerable pain and anxiety for patients, and a vast amount of lost sleep for junior doctors. However, their insertion is an important skill to acquire, and the ability to get one in quickly in a difficult situation can be life saving. You can't learn it from a book, but this chapter is a list of miscellaneous tips acquired over the years, which may be helpful in difficult cases.

Preparation

You need a decent tourniquet. One of the proper buckled variety, that allows you to increase the tension after it is applied, is best. The standard-issue green rubber NHS tourniquets are useless, and tend to be too short and pinch the skin. A sphygmomanometer inflated to 60–80 mmHg also works very well.

Always, **always** use local anaesthetic. Most of those young doctors waving 14-gauge venflons at old ladies have not had one inserted themselves. Believe me – they hurt. Lignocaine (1% without adrenaline) can be injected with a 25-gauge needle, or better still, with a diabetic syringe. None of the excuses for not using local is valid, and it basically all boils down to laziness. Injecting a bit of local only takes a few seconds, and if you find it more difficult with local, just practice until it becomes easier. If the bleb gets in the way, press on it for a second and it will disappear.

Apart from being more humane, local anaesthesia greatly reduces pain and anxiety, which means less vasoconstriction and better veins. If the first attempt is unsuccessful, then further tries can be made in a calmer atmosphere, without the escalating tension and anxiety that normally accompanies a multiple stabbing.

EMLA cream, a local anaesthetic preparation which has good transdermal absorption, can also be used. It is expensive, however, and must be applied under an occlusive dressing for at least an hour before it has a useful effect. It is mainly reserved for use in children, but can be used for those adults with genuine needle phobia.

For hairy patients, consider shaving the target area. This helps you to see the veins, helps to keep the drip in place, and is more comfortable for the patient when the dressing is removed.

Choose your weapon with care. Smaller gauge cannulae get progressively easier to insert, it's true. They also get progressively less useful; if rapid infusion is required, big is beautiful. If local anaesthetic is used, a 14-gauge (brown) is no more painful than a 20-gauge (pink). The final choice depends on the situation, but you had better have a jolly good reason for putting in anything smaller than an 18-gauge (green). Get in the habit of always wearing gloves. Blood should not be infused through anything smaller than an 18-gauge.

Choice of vein

In general, go for the vein you can feel, rather than the vein you can see. A suitable target vessel has an unmistakable springiness to touch as it is collapsed. Often, a big, fat-looking vein may be thrombosed, and non-springy. Excellent veins can be palpated in young chubby individuals where none can be seen. Avoid veins upstream of the site where a cannula has just tissued. Cannulae placed here will not last.

Of the available sites, the best are lateral distal forearm, or dorsum of hand. Choose the non-dominant side wherever possible. Having a cannula in the antecubital fossa is awkward, and sites which cross a joint are best avoided. Having said that, the antecubital fossa is the number one choice in times of crisis, particularly trauma and hypovolaemia, when a large bore cannula can be inserted rapidly. If none of these sites have suitable veins, the small veins on the anterior surface of the wrist will usually accept at least a 20-gauge. This is probably the most painful site, and hurts like mad even when local is used. The constant vein of Jenkins is a little-used vein that runs along the posteromedial aspect of the forearm and arm. It is best viewed with the elbow flexed upward. Don't forget that, with the exception of those on vascular surgery wards, most patients have an average of two legs. Feet and ankle veins are often good enough to use, although the incidence of thrombosis is reportedly greater. Don't forget also the cephalic vein in the upper arm, as it traverses biceps. This is a vein that is often better felt than seen. As a last resort, when all other veins are collapsed, the external jugular vein is often clearly visible.

Enhancement techniques

If there are no suitable veins available, the following may help.
- Tap the vein lightly with your fingers.
- Get help from gravity, let the arm dangle down below the level of the bed.
- Position a light to pass across the arm. This often demonstrates good veins by their shadows.
- Wait a few minutes with the tourniquet applied.
- Shove the patient's forearm in a jug of warm water for a minute or two.
- If you're really struggling, a GTN patch applied distal to the tourniquet works wonders (contraindications are aortic stenosis and hypovolaemia).
- If there is already a just-about-patent cannula *in situ*, infuse some fluid through it with a tourniquet applied. Other veins will become prominent.

Insertion

- When using a large-bore cannula, a small vertical skin incision made with the needle bevel facing to the side can help prevent the cannula being distorted as it passes through the skin.
- Turn the plastic cap of the injection port through 90° so that the hinge part points sideways. This gives you something to hold on to when you advance the cannula.
- Advancing the needle and cannula 1 mm after the 'flashback' is seen often makes threading more successful.
- Generally, advancing the cannula once under the skin shouldn't hurt. If it does, you are probably not in the vein. There should be negligible resistance to advancing the cannula.
- The cannula should be aimed proximally, that is *up* the arm, not down. (Don't laugh – it happened.)

Getting it to stay in

Much can be done to promote longevity in an i.v. cannula. Basically, they fail for two main reasons: they get pulled out or they 'tissue'.

Preventing dislodgement is down to choice of dressing. There are many different techniques that work, but any good dressing will prevent movement in a distal direction. If tinc. benz. spray is applied first, any kind of tape will stick much better. Put a loop in the giving set to prevent direct tension on the cannula. Circumferential dressings, that go right round an extremity, should be avoided. Occasionally with uncooperative patients, some ingenuity has to be used (e.g. setting the i.v. line in a plaster cast under anaesthesia).

Preventing a cannula 'tissuing' is more difficult. The more aseptic your technique the better, as infection plays a big role. Some drugs, such as penicillin or erythromycin, will very rapidly finish off any vein.

Other infusion problems

Avoid infusing dangerous drugs (for example insulin or morphine) into a drip with a three-way tap. There is a real risk that if the venflon tissues, the pump will go on infusing the wrong way up the tube. When you replace the venflon, the patient gets 500 units of insulin stat. Place a second smaller venflon (e.g. 22-gauge blue) for drugs, or use a specially designed antisiphon valve.

Alternatives to i.v. cannulae

It is worth remembering that in a crisis, effective therapy can often be given without a functioning i.v. cannula:
- Glucagon in hypoglycaemia can be given intramuscularly.
- Adrenaline in anaphylaxis can be given subcutaneously, or down the tracheal tube in cardiac arrest.
- Diazepam in status epilepticus can be given rectally.
- High-volume fluid resuscitation can be given through an intraosseous needle, a route particularly useful in children.
- A variety of drugs may be given by subcutaneous infusion. (See the Final Chapter for details.)

When to give up

Sooner or later, depending on experience, you will find yourself with a patient you can't cannulate. There are a number of options at this point. The first, soldiering on until you get it in, is not recommended. We think three tries for someone with less than average experience is plenty. The more you try, the more both patient and doctor are consumed with stress and anxiety, and the less likely you are to be successful. Furthermore, you are trashing veins that another person might successfully cannulate.

Secondly, you could call for help. The first port of call should always be your immediate superior. Do not call an anaesthetist straight away, unless you want to learn some new swear words. Many junior anaesthetists vehemently resist helping out with cannulae, for fear of eventually becoming a 'venflon service'. Personally, if asked I will have a go provided an SHO or registrar has also tried (and it's not the middle of the night). If all else fails, proceed to option three.

Thirdly, re-appraise the need for continued venous access. Any patient with difficult veins, who is likely to need venous access for a few more days, should be considered for a central line, or a Hickman line. Patients on long courses of i.v. antibiotics, especially penicillin or erythromycin, are especially worthy. An ordinary central line can be used for up to a week, a Hickman may last almost indefinitely, and both may also be used for drawing blood samples. They are reasonably comfortable when placed via the subclavian route, and do not hurt when inserted (provided local anaesthetic is used).

Chapter II.25

USING ITU

Using ITU

KEY POINTS

Use the ITU as a source of medical or nursing advice.
Keep in touch and visit your patients regularly.

Functions of ITU/HDU

Intensive Care or Intensive Therapy Units specialize in the treatment of patients with actual or potential life-threatening organ failure. Diverse surgical pathologies, when very severe, tend to follow a common path to multiple organ failure, which includes circulatory collapse, renal and ventilatory failure and DIC. To prevent this, or to deal with the results, ITUs collect a high level of nursing and medical expertise and specialized equipment. Such equipment includes mechanical ventilators, invasive monitors, haemodialysis or haemofiltration pumps and accurate infusion systems to control fluid and drug doses.

High Dependency Units care for somewhat less sick patients, rarely needing support of more than one organ system at a time. They are often sub-specialized to deal with particular pathologies (e.g. post-cardiac, postop recovery, burns and renal units).

Who needs ITU?

There is always competition for these specialized and expensive beds. Only patients with a realistic chance of meaningful recovery can be considered for a place, and these should require a greater level of care than can be expected from a general ward. Possibly the greatest benefit is gained by those in whom organ failure can be prevented by a short-term increase in the level of care (e.g. optimizing fluid balance after major abdominal surgery to avoid renal failure).

The following are indications to consider ITU for the surgical patient:

- Equipment needed beyond the expertise of the general ward; arterial lines, pulmonary artery catheters, intracranial pressure monitoring. In some hospitals epidurals and tracheostomies are only used on ITU/HDU.
- Requiring specialist organ support; ventilation, haemofiltration, TPN, cardiovascular support with inotropes or mechanical pumps.
- Patients at high risk of multiple organ failure (all influenced by pre-existing disease); sepsis, some cases of peritonitis, major trauma, burns.
- Patients requiring monitoring or observation beyond the scope of the general wards; neurological injuries, borderline renal, cardiovascular, respiratory function. Following major elective surgery.

Getting the most from ITU

Prevention is better than cure. If you are concerned about a patient, use ITU as a source of advice. ITU doctors should often be able to see your patient on the ward and may be able to help prevent a situation becoming critical. It is also important for the ITU staff to know about potential problem patients so that they can prioritize which of them most need admitting.

In major elective cases, ask ITU and the anaesthetist whether an admission is appropriate. Always check the ITU bed-state before these cases. Warn the ITU nurses as early as possible; they can often visit the patient preop to give reassurance and answer questions. Emergencies can be admitted to ITU preop to facilitate resuscitation.

Keep in touch. Surgical patients generally remain under the care of surgical consultants while they are in ITU. There will be technical questions for the surgeons to answer on wound care, splints, etc., and management decisions (e.g. regarding further surgery) to be made. As the house surgeon, you will be expected to act as liaison between ITU and your consultants. Unless you follow your ITU patients, you will also fail to understand their further management when they are discharged back to your care.

Keep a bed open. ITU must have the right to discharge patients at short notice if a more pressing case arrives. If you have an ITU patient who is within 1–2 days of discharge (which you will only know if you have visited the unit regularly), you must clear a bed for them.

The Final Chapter

DEATH

The Final Chapter

DEATH

KEY POINTS

Don't complain at the nurses when asked to declare death.
Death certificates may 'bounce' if they are not completed properly. Ask
the Coroner's advice when in doubt.
Inquests need not be too scary, particularly if you keep good notes.
Many doctors have no idea of the capabilities of modern palliative care
medicine. Expert advice is available to help you with the care of dying
patients.

Death: diagnosis

Don't laugh – mistakes are made regularly, resulting in great-aunt Hilda
waking up in a fridge. Death ought to be easy to diagnose, though severe
hypothermia or drug-induced coma may feature in the differential diagnosis.

It is a source of annoyance for house officers that they are called from their
beds to confirm death, but it is an unavoidable duty. The nursing staff cannot
make any further arrangements until death is confirmed. If, as in one famous
case, you tell the hapless nurses to do half-hourly neurological observations
and to call you in the event of a change, then you deserve everything you get
in return.

When called, you should shine a light in the eyes, and put a stethoscope on
the chest. Then you can write...

'No respiratory effort. Breath sounds/heart sounds – nil
Pupils fixed and dilated. Death confirmed at ...'

...and everyone's happy. (Well, you know what I mean.)

The death certificate

Provided there is no reason to refer the case to the Coroner (see below), you
can issue a death certificate. Use your best handwriting (and don't write in
pencil). It is usually required by the family the next day in order to make
funeral arrangements. Don't compound the grief of bereaved relatives by
keeping them hanging around for hours when they come to collect the
certificate.

Strictly speaking, the form you fill in (from the 'Celestial Chequebook') is
not the death certificate, but the medical certificate of cause of death. The
relatives take it to the Registrar of Deaths who will issue the true death
certificate.

The most important part of the form is the cause of death. You are invited
to give this as a chain of causes. Careful construction of this chain will avoid

The Final Chapter

problems. For example:

```
(Direct cause of death:)      1 a:  Left ventricular failure
(Caused by:)                    b:  Myocardial infarction
(Caused by:)                    c:  Ischaemic heart disease
(Contributory condition:)     2 :  Diabetes mellitus
```

...is acceptable.

Be aware that if your certificate is issued inappropriately, it will be 'bounced' by the Registrar, and referred to the Coroner. This can cause delay and distress to the relatives (and embarrassment to you) and can be avoided. Errors are of two types:

1. When a certificate is issued where the case should have been referred to the Coroner. For example:

```
1a: Brain haemorrhage
 b: Gunshot wound to the head
```

or...

```
1a: Bronchopneumonia
 b: Fractured neck of femur
 c: Being pushed out of a window by her son
2 : Gross lifelong neglect by her vile family
```

...are likely to bounce. The full list of indications for referral to the Coroner is given below, but anything suggestive of trauma, neglect or unnatural death should always be referred.

2. When the cause of death is not given clearly, or is worded in such a way as to raise a doubt in the mind of the Registrar, who is a lay person. For example:

```
1a: Heart failure
```

or:

```
1a: Sepsis
```

...may not give adequate information. Everyone's heart stops when they die. If you have evidence that heart failure was due to ischaemic heart disease or myocardial infarction, say so in parts 1b and 1c. Another example is death due to 'cerebrovascular accident', which to a layman suggests either trauma or medical mishap, both of which would be Coroner's cases.

In many cases the Coroner will allow a 'bounced' certificate to pass after discussion with the doctor concerned.

It is helpful to write the cause of death in the notes, as written on the Medical Certificate.

The Coroner

The first Coroners were all knights appointed in 1194 by Richard I. Their original task was as revenue officers. Investigation of death was only part of their duties, and even then the emphasis was on finding out what *article* caused the death. By the process of 'Deodand', the offending object (e.g. a cart) was confiscated and sold.

These days, the Coroner can be a lawyer or a doctor, and is occasionally both. The Coroner's court is fundamentally different from other judicial courts in that it is *inquisitorial* rather than *accusatorial*. A Coroner's job is to establish the facts surrounding a death, and not to apportion blame.

The Coroner is responsible ultimately to the Home Secretary, and not the Lord Chancellor like other judicial officers. Appeals against his verdicts have to be heard at the High Court.

Cases that should be referred to the coroner are:

- Deaths occurring within 24 h of admission.
- When the attending doctor did not see the deceased within 14 days before or after death. (Unlikely in hospital, I hope.)
- Deaths occurring under anaesthesia, or within 24 h of an operation. There is no statutory requirement to keep people alive for this time, as some seem to believe.
- Deaths as a result of trauma of any kind. This includes fractured femur in the elderly.
- Deaths attributable to alcohol.
- Deaths due to medical mishaps. In this instance it is in the best interests of the doctor concerned for the Coroner to handle the case.
- Deaths resulting from industrial diseases, for example pneumoconiosis.
- Where the doctor is unsure as to the cause of death.
- Deaths resulting from violence or neglect.

It is important to note that the coroner does not necessarily have to order a post-mortem examination, and in many cases the medical certificate can be issued at the Coroner's discretion. If there is *any* doubt, it is much better to ask the Coroner for advice, rather than issue a dud certificate. Coroners also vary in their opinions, so that for example 'cerebrovascular accident' is acceptable in some districts and not others. When in doubt *ask*.

Inquests

There are circumstances when the Coroner is obliged to hold an inquest. The most common examples are: any case of sudden and unnatural death, trauma, suicides, unexpected deaths in hospital and deaths under anaesthesia.

During an inquest, the Coroner will hear evidence from relevant parties, including doctors. If called, you will be asked to write a report, and you will be questioned on it. Remember, although it may feel very much like you are on trial, the Coroner is *not* seeking to apportion blame, he merely wants the facts. In many cases (e.g. death during surgery for ruptured aneurysm), an inquest is simply a legal formality, and nothing to feel threatened by.

All sorts of people have a right to ask questions at an inquest, so do not be surprised if you are cross-examined by a lawyer representing an insurance company or an employer.

Tips which may help:

- Stick to facts when answering questions. Avoid opinions.
- The vast majority of sticky moments at inquests are the fault of poor note keeping. Think of the poor casualty SHO who had to explain to the court

what his entry 'T.T.F.O' in the notes meant[a]. This and other such jokey entries (NFN = 'Normal for Norfolk', FUBARD BUNDY= 'Fouled Up Beyond All Reasonable Doubt But Unfortunately Not Dead Yet', PBAB KLO ='Pine Box at Bedside – Keep Lid Open) tend to lose their comedy value in a court full of wailing relatives. You may find it hard to answer detailed questions if you made no entries in the notes for a week before death.

- Read the notes carefully beforehand. Refer to your report when giving evidence.
- Arrange a meeting with health authority lawyers beforehand. Many trusts now have Risk Management departments, who will go through the case with you and offer specific advice. Often the trust itself will be legally represented at the inquest. If you are a member of a defence organization, they can offer advice. (If you aren't, you should be.)

The cremation form

The cremation form is a document that legally releases the deceased's remains for cremation. It was designed at the turn of the century, and is a statutory form (i.e. it requires an act of parliament to change the wording. This explains some of the arcane questions). When you sign a cremation form, it boils down to staking your reputation on three facts:
1. That the cause of death is certain.
2. That you are not mentioned in the deceased's will.
3. That the deceased will not explode or cause radioactive fallout when cremated, due to a pacemaker or radioactive implant.

There is also a registrar at the crematorium who can bounce the form if there is a problem, though this is very rare.

You probably know that a useful wad of cash is paid for signing the form. The Inland Revenue knows this, too. Resist attempts by parsimonious SHOs to 'claim' your ash cash as public property, to fund the doctor's mess or such like. The mess should be funded by all who use it. Housemen are paid less than anyone else; crem forms are your *only* perk.

Talking to relatives and generally giving bad news

Telling people that their relative is dead or dying, or telling patients they have an incurable condition is a difficult task for which we receive no training. The following tips were all gained from bitter experience.

First of all, if you have bad news, make time to tell it properly. It is no good rushing in, saying how sorry you are, and then dashing off to an X-ray meeting. Choose a private area where you can all sit down, and always, always have a nurse with you. Someone has to pick up the pieces after you've gone.

Be aware of your body language. Maintain eye contact. It is amazing how many doctors inadvertently smile – an instinctive response to nervousness. If you are dealing with a large and close family, identify a spokesperson to avoid having to speak to every member in turn.

Most people will either not remember a thing you say (hence the need for simplicity and directness), or will remember your *exact words* for the rest of

[a] According to the story he said it meant 'Told To Follow Orders'. Full marks for thinking on your feet!

their lives, so make it good. Be honest (though not brutal), and for goodness' sake avoid clichés or euphemisms. "Going to a better place" may be interpreted as being transferred to another hospital. If you think a patient is dying, say so. Don't overload the audience with information that they would not understand at the best of times. Whilst remaining broadly truthful, offer comforts such as "he didn't suffer" or "we will continue to keep him comfortable", but don't go overboard.

Be prepared for the questions that everyone asks, but no-one can answer. "How long?", "What are the chances of survival?" If, however, you are ignorant of basic facts of the case, you shouldn't be there. Never be drawn into hypothetical discussions, for example "If our GP had come out sooner, would he have survived?"

Afterwards, ask for feedback from the accompanying nurse. Most experienced nurses have seen hundreds of these interviews, and will be able to help you improve your performance next time. (Make no mistake – you are performing.) If one of your seniors is giving the news, don't be shut out – go and watch.

Finally, it helps others if you write in the patient's notes that the interview took place, and roughly what was said.

Bereavement counselling has been shown to be highly effective when offered to relatives in the weeks following the loss. It can help to prevent disabling psychiatric problems that might otherwise affect many members of the extended family. The commonest problems for relatives are inappropriate feelings of guilt. Many hospitals now offer such a support system which is usually based around the ITU.

Brain death and organ donation

This is only ever an ITU concern, but patient's relatives sometimes ask about donation anyway. Organs are only any use if they are still being perfused at the time of harvest, and are thus only retrieved from ventilated, brain-dead intensive care unit patients.

Euthanasia

Euthanasia is illegal, although it undoubtedly occurs. A doctor was recently convicted of attempted murder for injecting a patient with potassium chloride to end her suffering.

Changes in the law have been resisted for both moral and practical reasons, (i.e. "do we have the right?" and "can we stop any system being abused?"). The majority of doctors polled are in favour of legalization of euthanasia. You may be surprised to learn that when the doctors polled are specialists in palliative care or pain relief, the proportion in favour is dramatically less.

There is, unfortunately, widespread ignorance of the capabilities of modern palliative care medicine. Euthanasia poses serious ethical questions, but in many cases it may simply be unnecessary.

Terminal care

Terminally ill patients occasionally appear on surgical wards, often as the result of an emergency admission, and an 'open and close' laparotomy, or when admitted for investigations that uncover inoperable malignancies. Management of such patients, when everyone else has lost interest, usually falls to the person with the least experience, that is you.

Symptom control thus becomes the only concern, so unpleasant techniques and procedures normally intended to prolong life become unnecessary. Effective control of distressing symptoms can be achieved without venflons, nasogastric tubes or intramuscular injections. The most common problems are pain, nausea and vomiting, bowel obstruction, 'rattle', thrush and constipation.

Pain

The usual principles of pain relief apply, but with a few extra considerations. Opioids are usually required, but try to use the oral route wherever possible. This avoids dependence on needles. The opioid of choice is morphine elixir (Oramorph®), which is given 4-hourly. The idea is to increase the dose every 4 h until pain is controlled. When a stable dose is achieved, divide the total dose in 24 h by two, and give it as MST twice a day.

If parenteral therapy is required, the most commonly used drug is diamorphine. Avoid short-acting drugs like pethidine. Please note that it does not have to be intravenous (see below). The correct dose is **as much as is required to relieve pain**. Do not approach these problems with pre-conceived ideas about the 'correct dose' of diamorphine. Start treatment for nausea and vomiting and constipation at the same time (see below).

There are, however, some forms of pain which do not respond to opioids, and such patients need to be identified, as there are other measures which may help them:

- Bone pain, from metastases, responds well to non-steroidal anti-inflammatory drugs, and very well to radiotherapy. Often a single visit to a radiotherapy unit will bring dramatic relief. Non-steroidals are a useful adjunct in all forms of pain.
- Raised intracranial pressure from intracerebral metastases often responds to dexamethasone.
- Muscle spasm may respond to diazepam or baclofen.
- Neurogenic pain, as suggested by symptoms of lancinating (shooting) pains or excessive sensitivity to touch may respond to carbamazepine, baclofen or amitriptyline.
- In difficult cases, where pain is anywhere below the nipples, do not be afraid to ask an anaesthetist about an epidural.

PRN = 'pain relief non-existent'. Choose a regimen of **regular** medication.

Nausea and vomiting

The management of nausea and vomiting in malignancy differs slightly from perioperative emesis. Many different factors may be involved, and the palliative care approach is to identify the most likely cause, and treat accordingly.

- Gut-related vomiting, from gastric irritation, abdominal carcinoma or intestinal obstruction, is best treated with metoclopramide 10–20 mg tds subcutaneously.
- Chemoreceptor trigger zone-related vomiting, from drugs (opioids), biochemical disorders or toxins, is best treated with an antidopaminergic drug. The favoured agent in terminal care is haloperidol 2.5–5 mg

subcutaneously.
- Vomiting related to higher centres (i.e. fear and anxiety), or raised intracranial pressure, can be managed with diazepam, 2–10 mg.
- Vestibular apparatus-related sickness can be treated with hyoscine, 0.4 mg subcutaneously or with a transdermal patch ('Scopaderm').
- Unknown cause, or for add-on therapy, use cyclizine 50 mg tds subcutaneously.

Bowel obstruction
Many terminally ill patients die in bowel obstruction, and much can be done to alleviate the symptoms. Principles of management are:
- Analgesia, usually diamorphine.
- Anti-emetics, haloperidol 5 mg and cyclizine 150 mg, by subcutaneous infusion (see below). A realistic aim is to keep vomiting to once a day or less.
- For colic, add hyoscine 60–120 mg daily.
- Second line treatment, try octreotide 300 mcg daily by subcutaneous infusion, instead of hyoscine. This is a relatively new (and expensive) drug which acts in a similar way to somatostatin, and 'switches off' secretion and motility in the gut. It can sometimes have a dramatic effect on abdominal distension.
- Nasogastric tubes and i.v. fluids are **not necessary**.

Death rattle
This is caused by chest secretions. Try hyoscine 30–80 mg by syringe driver, or 20 mg subcutaneously. Established rattle is difficult to treat, and may require gentle suctioning or careful positioning of the patient.

Oral thrush
This is common and difficult to treat. Fluconazole is more effective than nystatin.

Constipation
Use a combination of softener and stimulant (e.g. co-danthramer), unless there is bowel obstruction, in which case use a pure softener (e.g. docusate).

Other measures
- Go through the drug chart, and ditch anything that has no palliative value.
- Consider draining pleural effusions or ascites where they are causing discomfort.
- Consider parenteral therapy by subcutaneous infusion. For this you need a small, portable syringe driver that takes a 10-ml syringe (e.g. Graseby MS26 or MS16). A 24-h dose of the drug is made up to 10 ml and infused through a butterfly placed under the skin in the upper chest or abdomen. Drugs which can be infused include diamorphine, cyclizine, haloperidol, metoclopramide, midazolam, octreotide and hyoscine. Butterflies need to be resited every 48 h or so to prevent inflammation, unless the infusion is diamorphine alone when it will last for 2 weeks or more. Swelling or soreness will respond to a daily dose of dexamethasone 1 mg. Drugs *not* to use subcutaneously are chlorpromazine,

prochlorperazine or diazepam.

Finally, in difficult cases, do not hesitate to ask for advice. Some or all of the following should be available locally:

- Hospital Palliative Care support team.
- Hospital Macmillan Nurse.
- Breast care nurse.
- Local hospice.
- Pain clinic.

Action plan for
ANALGESIC DRUGS

The values given are for suggested maintenance dosages.
These figures are for the entirely fictional healthy 70-kg adult.
All patients need to be *loaded* first (see Chapter II.3).
You may need to give *more* if the patient is young and muscular,
or less if they are small, elderly, or suffering from cardiovascular
or renal disease.
The only way to be sure is to titrate and reassess.

Morphine

- Intermittent i.m. injection 10–15 mg 3-hourly.
- Intravenous loading dose: increments of 2.5–5 mg at 5-min intervals.
- Intravenous infusion: draw up 50 mg in 50 ml, and run at 3–5 ml/h initially. If pain returns give a small loading dose as well as increasing the infusion rate.
- Patient-controlled analgesia: typically 1-mg bolus, lockout 5 min.
- Oral: morphine elixir start at 5–10 mg every 4 h, and increase the dose each time until control is achieved. When comfortable, multiply the 4-hourly dose by three and give as MST every 12 h.

Pethidine

- Intermittent i.m. injection: 75–100 mg 2-hourly PRN.
- Intravenous loading dose: increments of 25 mg at 5-min intervals.
- Intravenous infusion: draw up 500 mg in 50 ml and give 3–5 ml/h initially. Beware norpethidine toxicity at doses over 1000 mg per day. If doses approaching this level are required, consider using a different drug.
- Patient-controlled analgesia: 10-mg bolus, lockout 5 min.
- Oral: don't.

Diamorphine

- Intermittent i.m. injection 5–10 mg 3-hourly.
- Intravenous loading dose: increments of 1–2 mg at 3-min intervals.
- Intravenous infusion: 50 mg in 50 ml at a rate of 1–3 ml/h.
- Patient-controlled analgesia: 0.5 mg bolus, lockout 3 min.
- Oral: no advantage over oral morphine.

(continued)

Action plan for
ANALGESIC DRUGS
(continued)

Agent	Route	Equipotent dose (mg)	Onset (min)	Duration (h)	Dose interval (h)
Morphine	i.m.	10	15	4	3–4
	i.v.	5	5	3–4	
elixir:	Oral	30	30	4	4
slow release:	Oral	30	240	12	12
Pethidine	i.m.	100	15	3	
	i.v.	50	5	2	3
	Oral	300	120		
Diamorphine	i.m.	5	30	3	3–4
	i.v.	2.5	15		
Fentanyl	i.v.	0.1	1	0.5–1	
Methadone	i.m.	10	30	5	6–12
	Oral	20	120	4	
Codeine	i.m.	120	20	4	4–6
	Oral	200			

Action plan for
ANAPHYLAXIS

Suggested by: urticaria and flushing with hypotension, broncho-spasm, or glottic oedema, particularly if after an i.v. injection.

1. ABCs: airway, oxygen, venous access, crash team. Discontinue suspected drugs.
2. Adrenaline, 0.1 mg (1 ml of 1 in 10 000 as in Minijet) i.v., repeated as necessary.
3. ECG monitoring.
4. Rapid i.v. fluid therapy (e.g. a litre of saline stat).
5. Glottic oedema poses a serious airway risk, which may need urgent management.
6. Bronchospasm that persists after the acute episode should be treated with aminophylline 5 mg/kg i.v. over 30 min.
7. Second-line therapy: chlorpheniramine (Piriton) 10–20 mg i.v. slowly, hydrocortisone 200 mg i.v.

Take two EDTA blood samples. Speak to an immunologist about further investigation. Document the event and suspected drug fully.

Action plan for
ACUTE ASTHMA

1. Assess for danger signs (silent chest, inability to speak, cyanosis, extreme tachycardia). If any are present, call ITU or medical registrar. Order blood gases. Check X-ray for pneumothorax.
2. Give humidified oxygen, try not to panic.
3. Give salbutamol nebulizer 2.5 ml stat. Repeat **as often as necessary.**
4. Give hydrocortisone 200 mg i.v. and repeat 4-hourly.
5. Avoid sedatives, get help from anaesthetics if acute pain co-exists.
6. If continued deterioration, aminophylline can be given 250 mg i.v., but if you have got this far it is **definitely** time to seek expert help (i.e. medical registrar or ITU).
7. Rapidly rising P_aCO_2 is an indication for ventilation.
8. Bradycardia is an indication to call the crash team.

Action plan for
ATRIAL FIBRILLATION

Suggested by rapid (120–180 b.p.m.) irregular, narrow-complex tachycardia, with no P waves.

1. Basic life support: airway, breathing, oxygen, venous access, finger on pulse, blood pressure.
2. If shocked, get help fast. The patient may require urgent cardioversion under general anaesthesia.
3. Check potassium. Look for possible cause, pulmonary embolus, hypoxia, myocardial infarction, pain, hypovolaemia.
4. For the undigitalized patient, once you have excluded hypokalaemia, give digoxin 500 mcg orally, followed by one or two further doses at 6-hourly intervals. Give maintenance therapy as 250 mcg daily. Loading doses can be given orally. Reduce the maintenance dose in the elderly or in renal impairment.
5. If the patient takes digoxin already, and has a normal serum potassium, give a single dose of 500 mcg.
6. Check digoxin levels at the earliest opportunity.

Action plan for
BLEEDING

1. Control bleeding: elevation, direct pressure, pressure on artery. No tourniquets, clips.
2. Establish good i.v. access (14- or 16-gauge) away from bleeding site. Send FBC, coagulation, U&E, cross-match. Start charting vital signs at 15-min intervals. Use signs to estimate loss and guide treatment. Give initial fluid resuscitation immediately as a bolus:

   - Pulse 100+, systolic BP normal, diastolic raised, urine 30+ ml/h:
     loss 750+
       salt solution 1000–1500 ml, or colloid 350–500 ml.
   - Pulse 120+, systolic BP low, diastolic low, urine <30 ml/h, confused:
     loss 1500+
       salt solution 1000–2000 ml, or colloid 500–1000 ml, plus blood 2 units.
   - Pulse 140+, systolic low, diastolic low, no urine, lethargic:
     loss 2000+
       salt solution 1000–2000 ml, or colloid 500–1000 ml plus blood 4 units (consider FFP/platelets).

3. Get help. Senior surgeon needed in all cases. Anaesthetist and theatres for re-explorations. ITU and haematology for coagulopathy.
4. Move to safer place. Provide O_2. Catheterize. Keep warm with blood-warmer and hot air blanket (may need to borrow these from theatre).
5. Review drugs. Discontinue NSAID, heparin, warfarin. Discontinue i.m. drug route.
6. After initial resuscitation (above), review vital signs and lab results. Give platelets if count <100; FFP if INR >2.0; blood to keep [Hb] at 10.
7. Continue fluids until urine output is >0.5 ml/kg/h, normal level of consciousness, tachycardia and hypotension resolving.
8. Platelets and FFP are likely to be needed after 6–8 units of blood, but be guided by repeated lab tests.
9. Arrange transfer to receive definitive care (theatres or ITU). Maintain fluids, O_2, monitoring and temperature in transfer.

Action plan for
BLEEDING IN CHILDREN

1. Principles as for adults.
2. Vital signs differ: normal pulse higher, BP lower, urine output higher. Early signs of shock are reduced skin perfusion and tachycardia.
3. Total blood volume is 8% of weight.
4. Initial bolus for fluid resuscitation in shock is **20 ml/kg.**
5. Repeat bolus only after careful re-evaluation of signs.
6. If bleeding exceeds 25 ml/kg (30% of blood volume), or shock persists transfuse with blood boluses of **10 ml/kg.** *Warm all fluids with an approved device.*

Action plan for
DIABETIC KETOACIDOSIS

1. Inform surgeons, anaesthetist and ITU.
2. Establish large-bore i.v., nasogastric tube, urinary catheter and oxygen.
3. Move to observation area, start charts and ECG monitoring. 15 min obs and urine output.
4. Send baseline tests: U&E, gases, glucose, FBC.
5. Fluid resuscitation: 0.9% saline + KCl 20 mmol/l at 2 l/h initially.
6. Bolus dose insulin: Actrapid 20 units i.v.
7. Start insulin infusion: Actrapid 10 units/h.
8. Repeat U&E, gases, glucose very frequently (half-hourly). ITU analyser may be quicker than laboratory.
9. Replace glucose as it falls below 10 mmol/l: dextrose 10% 100 ml/h.
10. pH<7.0, consider bicarbonate, but talk to ITU first.
11. All cases need ITU referral.

Action plan for
EXTRAPYRAMIDAL SIDE-EFFECTS (EPSEs)

Caused by the antidopaminergic effects of many commonly used anti-emetics and major tranquillizers, for example metoclopramide ('Maxolon'), Prochlorperazine ('Stemetil'), droperidol, chlorpromazine, haloperidol and others.

EPSEs are more common in young women. Typical signs are motor restlessness (akathisia) also known as 'the jitters', leading to a wide range of involuntary dystonic movements, especially of the face and neck. Lip smacking, eye-rolling (oculogyric crisis) and ballistic movements of the limbs may occur. The patient remains fully conscious.

Management: give procyclidine 5 mg i.m., repeated after 10 min if necessary. Discontinue any of the drugs mentioned above. Write up cyclizine 50 mg 8-hourly i.m. for nausea.

Action plan for
HYPERKALAEMIA

Serum potassium greater than 6.0 needs treatment. Acute hyperkalaemia is much more dangerous than chronic.

1. 10 ml of 10% calcium gluconate i.v. slowly.
2. If there is acidosis, correct it. Give 8.4% bicarbonate

    volume of 8.4% bicarbonate (ml) = base deficit x body weight (kg) x 0.3

    Give half the calculated dose initially.
3. Give dextrose and insulin, for example 50 ml of 50% dextrose with 20 units of soluble insulin over 30 min.
    None of these measures removes potassium from the body. To do this either:
4. Give calcium resonium 30 g t.i.d. orally or rectal, or
5. Arrange dialysis, for acute renal failure.

Action plan for
HYPOGLYCAEMIA

BM <4
1. Stop any insulin.
2. If oral route available: half pint of milk with 4–5 spoonsful of sugar.
3. If not: set up i.v. with 10% dextrose at 100 ml/h.
4. Check BM sticks hourly.

BM <2.5
1. If i.v. available: give 25 ml of 50% dextrose and reassess CNS function.
2. If still aggressive or comatose repeat step 1.
3. Check BM stix.
4. If no i.v: give i.m. glucagon 1 mg.
5. Check BM sticks half-hourly.
6. Significant insulin overdose may need ITU for central venous access, monitoring, cardiovascular and metabolic support.

Action plan for
HYPOTENSION

1. Ensure a clear airway, make sure there is breathing, give oxygen.
2. Check the pulse for rate and character. Insert a large i.v. cannula, put up some normal saline. Check for visible bleeding (e.g. from drains, etc.). If there is significant bleeding, call a surgeon.
3. If there has been a sudden, dramatic deterioration call the crash team. Consider mechanical cause, for example tension pneumothorax.
4. If the patient is awake and talking, proceed with detailed assessment. Begin by taking the BP yourself, manually.
5. Review the history, particularly recent fluid history. Full clinical examination by systems.
6. Review or order investigations. FBC, U&E, blood for cross-match. ECG, CXR if clinically indicated. Consider urinary catheter, and/or CVP line.
7. Unless good clinical evidence of cardiogenic shock (tachypnoea, raised JVP, gallop rhythm, poor peripheral perfusion), give 250 ml of normal saline, stat. If there is obvious haemorrhage use **warmed** blood.

Re-evaluate, and, if things have improved slightly, repeat as often as necessary to restore haemodynamic stability, reassessing at every stage. If things get worse with a fluid challenge, consider non-hypovolaemic aetiology. This usually means senior assistance.

Action plan for 'ILL'

Quite often, you will be called by an experienced nurse to see a patient who they feel is 'not quite right'. Take this warning very seriously indeed. In the absence of specific clues, you may need to follow a checklist in order to exclude life-threatening pathologies, and to identify the dangerously ill patient, for whom senior assistance is required.

If you keep the following headings in mind when called to see a non-specifically ill patient, you are unlikely to miss important pathologies, and you will have accumulated the relevant information for discussion with more senior doctors.

1. Systems-based assessment:
   - General state: colour, temperature (high or low), hydration, wound.
   - Cardiovascular system: pulse, blood pressure, urine output.
   - Respiratory system: rate (high or low), cyanosis or oximeter reading, auscultation.
   - Gut: distension, pain, ileus.
   - CNS: delirium, depressed consciousness, pain, agitation.

2. Review drug chart.

3. Investigations
   - Full blood count, urea and electrolytes, glucose, blood gases, ECG.

4. Supportive management in all cases:
   - oxygen therapy;
   - increased level of observation, monitoring devices as appropriate;
   - venous access;
   - get the appropriate level of advice or help.

Action plan for
INSULIN REGIMENS

Sliding scale insulin. Glucose is provided independently of the insulin as an i.v. infusion (dextrose 10% + KCl 20 mmol/l at 100 ml/h). Insulin is provided i.v. at a rate determined by the BM stick results. The normal insulin production is ~2 units per hour, so make 2 units/h correspond to the target blood glucose. Some diabetics are insulin resistant and routinely take much higher daily doses. Simply add up all their daily insulin and divide the number of units by 24 to get the hourly insulin dose which should correspond to the target blood glucose. Then range the insulin dose against the BM stick results. For example:

Glucose	Units insulin/h
<4	0 Call doctor
4.1–7.0	1
7.1–10	2 Target range
10.1–13	3
13.1–17	4
>17	Call doctor

Be sure to add instructions to call a doctor at either extreme of the range and on how often to measure the glucose (usually 1–2 h intervals). Insulin controls potassium flux into cells and serum K^+ will need checking regularly (every 12 h).

Alberti regime. In an attempt to simplify this, insulin, glucose and potassium are given together in a fixed ratio:

500 ml dextrose 10% + Actrapid 10 units + KCl 10 mmol.

Run this at a rate of 100 ml/h and check the BM stick every 2 h. If the glucose falls below 5 mmol/l, put up a new bag containing less insulin (6 units Actrapid). If the glucose rises above 10 mmol/l put up a new bag with more insulin (14 units Actrapid). As above, keep a close eye on the potassium.

Action plan for
OLIGURIA

1. Refer to notes for evidence of chronic renal impairment.
2. Examine with reference to volume status and urinary obstruction.
3. Catheterize and change to buretted collection system.
4. Chart hourly urine output and vital signs.
5. Fluid challenge: gelatin solution 200 ml and review, repeat if no improvement.
6. If no response, consider need for central line.
7. Titrate fluid until CVP has increased by 5 cmH_2O, unless initial reading is greater than 15 cmH_2O.
8. If no response, exclude ARF; send urine and blood for osmolarity and electrolytes.
9. Refer all cases of ARF to ITU or renal unit.
10. If oliguric with high CVP but not in ARF, consider dopamine and ITU referral.
11. All cases: prevent hypoxia and review drugs for nephrotoxins.

Action plan for
PREOPERATIVE INVESTIGATIONS

Few screening tests are valuable because of the low pick-up rate, exceptions are urinalysis and blood pressure measurement. These are essential in every case. Only directly relevant tests should be ordered and **if a test is worth ordering the result is worth looking at**. Here are some rough guidelines for testing:

FBC

>Age 60 or greater
>Anticipated blood loss >250 ml
>History or signs to suggest bleeding tendency, blood loss or anaemia
>Any known haematological illness
>Any significant connective tissue/autoimmune disease
>Any significant respiratory, cardiovascular, hepatic or renal disease
>Malnutrition or cachexia

Electrolytes/urea/creatinine

>Renal disease
>Patients with i.v. rehydration therapy (recent result)
>Diuretic, steroid, antidysrhythmic drugs
>Urinary outflow obstruction
>Age 60 or greater
>Significant cardiovascular, hepatic, endocrine (including diabetes) disease

Clotting studies

>Clinical suspicion of bleeding tendency
>Anti-coagulation
>Hepatic disease

Glucose

>Diabetes
>Steroid therapy

(continued)

Action plan for
PREOPERATIVE INVESTIGATIONS
(Continued)

Sickledex
> African and West-Indian ethnic groups. Follow all positive results with electrophoresis

ECG
> Age 60 or greater
> Age 40 or greater with a strong smoking history
> Any significant history or signs of cardiovascular disease in any age group
> Moderate/severe respiratory disease
> Severe connective tissue disease

CXR
> Very rarely indicated
> Possible metastases and infectious disease (TB) in high-risk populations
> Patients with severe or worsening cardiorespiratory illness, unless recent radiographs already exist
> Correctable lesions identified by clinical examination: pneumothorax, effusions, abscesses, pulmonary oedema

Viral illness
> Hepatitis B serology in:
> - liver disease
> - unexplained jaundice
> - drug abuse
> - prison inmates
> - male homosexuals
> - travellers from Africa, India and S. America

HIV screening must not be undertaken without the patient's permission and without support counselling. Antiviral protection should be used for **all** cases and not just those who appear to be at high risk.

Action plan for
PULMONARY OEDEMA

Dyspnoea, sweating, frothy sputum, gallop rhythm, raised venous pressure, basal crepitations.

1. Sit up, give oxygen, measure blood pressure. Get help if hypotensive.
2. Give morphine i.v., 2.5–10 mg in divided doses.
3. Give frusemide 20–40 mg i.v.
4. Identify and treat dysrhythmias (with a 12-lead ECG), rule out acute myocardial infarction.
5. Consider vasodilators if the blood pressure is good enough (e.g. isosorbide dinitrate 2–10 mg/h).
6. For severe respiratory distress or hypotension, consider transfer to ICU.

Action plan for
REFRACTORY NAUSEA AND VOMITING

1. Give up using metoclopramide routinely.
2. Give appropriate i.v. fluids (with potassium), consider nasogastric tube, check urea and electrolytes.
3. Take a history, examine, order relevant investigations looking for treatable underlying causes (e.g. bowel obstruction, acute abdomen, pancreatitis).
4. Review recent anti-emetic therapy.
5. If no anti-emetics have been given recently, start with pro-chlorperazine 12.5 mg i.m.
6. If an antidopaminergic drug (metoclopramide, prochlorperazine, droperidol, chlorpromazine or haloperidol) has been used within 6 h don't try any other antidopaminergic drugs. It is unlikely to be effective and you run a serious risk of causing a dystonic reaction. Try one (or a combination) of the following:
   - cyclizine 50 mg i.m.
   - ondansetron 4 mg i.v.
   - hyoscine 0.2 mg i.m.

Action plan for
RESPIRATORY DISTRESS

1. *Monitoring*: regular blood gases, pulse oximeter, daily CXR.
2. *Oxygen therapy*: controlled or otherwise.
3. *Exclude a pneumothorax*. They don't respond to bronchodilators.
4. *Remove all impediments to breathing* as far as possible. Sit up. Relieve abdominal distension, avoid tight circumferential dressings, avoid sedatives.
5. *Adequate analgesia*: contact anaesthetics or acute pain team for help.
6. *Control of sputum:* physiotherapy, postural drainage. Tracheal suction via minitracheostomy if drowning in sputum.
7. *Control of bronchospasm*. When in doubt, ask medical registrar.
8. *Control of infection*. Blood/sputum cultures. Early microbiological advice.
9. *Control of lung water*. If CXR evidence of oedema, careful fluid balance, diuretics.
10. *Control of right heart failure.*
11. *Losing the battle?* Inform ITU sooner rather than later.

Action plan for
SUPERVENTRICULAR TACHYCARDIA (SVT)

SVT is overdiagnosed. Many cases are in fact atrial fibrillation, sinus tachycardia or atrial flutter. SVT is a regular, narrow-complex tachycardia with a rate of 140–250. Many patients have a history of paroxysmal palpitations.

1. Exclude sinus tachycardia, atrial fibrillation, atrial flutter and their respective causes.
2. Try physiological manoeuvres. Carotid sinus massage or sustained Valsalva (blow into a sphygmomanometer tube to a pressure of 20 mmHg for 10 sec).
3. If this fails, try adenosine 3 mg slowly i.v., with ECG monitoring. If this has no effect after 1–2 min, give 6 mg, then 12 mg. Adenosine causes flushing, and transient hypotension that can be severe.
4. If this fails, the commonest reason is wrong diagnosis (for example sinus tachycardia). Some patients require DC cardioversion under general anaesthesia.

Action plan for
VENTRICULAR TACHYCARDIA

Any broad-complex tachycardia is VT until proven otherwise.

1. Immediate basic life support: airway, breathing, oxygen, venous access, feel the pulse. If absent call a cardiac arrest. Defibrillate with 200 J.
2. If good volume pulse, call for help and do a 12-lead ECG. Differential diagnosis is tachycardia in the presence of bundle branch block.
3. If confirmed VT give 100 mg of lignocaine i.v. (5 ml of 2%).
4. Follow with an infusion at 1–4 mg/h.
5. Check electrolytes, consider transfer to CCU or ICU.

INDEX